Diabetes A to Z

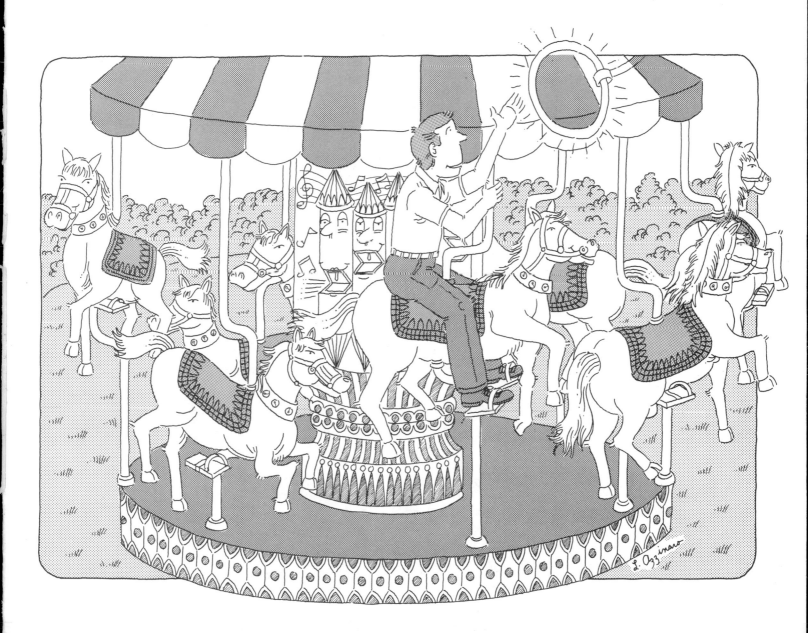

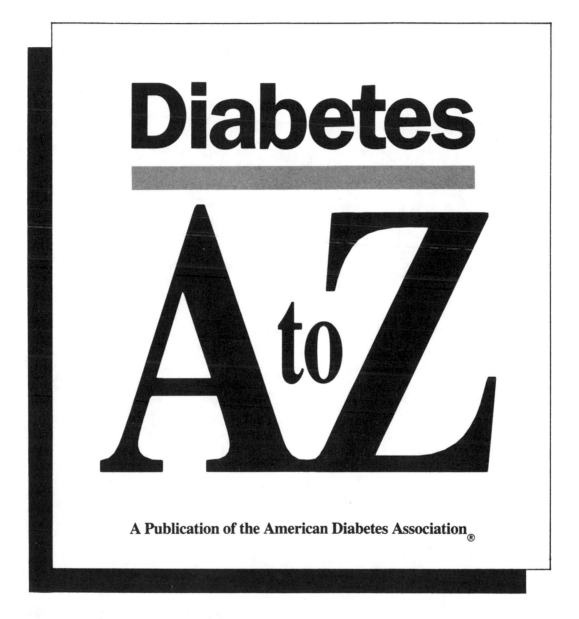

Diabetes

A to Z

A Publication of the American Diabetes Association®

Illustrations by Lew Azzinaro

ISBN 0-945448-03-1

Preface

Diabetes A to Z draws on the American Diabetes Association's 50-year tradition of excellence in providing high-quality information to people with diabetes and those who care for them. *Diabetes A to Z* is an expanded and updated version of the former *Guide to Good Living*. This book is meant to provide current information that will help those who have diabetes and encourage them to live the best life possible.

In *Diabetes A to Z*, we've particularly emphasized ways to integrate good diabetes management into a vigorous lifestyle. We've tried to focus on the healthy, energetic life—one that includes good nutrition, regular exercise, closer relationships with family and friends, a positive outlook on the present, and realistic hopes for the future. The individual with diabetes can and should participate in this full, vibrant lifestyle, not only because participation can mean better control and better health, but because it can be enriching, satisfying, and *fun*!

Diabetes A to Z has been organized like a dictionary, but it is unlike any ordinary dictionary. Not only are the entries longer, but each focuses on some aspect of living with diabetes. This publication is meant to be browsed through, to be picked up when you have a specific question, and to be used to revive your enthusiasm when you're feeling low. Also, it is important to note that this book is not limited to the person who has diabetes; those who don't have diabetes, but who live or work with someone who does, can benefit from the information contained in *Diabetes A to Z*.

We hope you will enjoy this book. But, more important, we hope this information will help you manage your diabetes so that your life can be happier and more fulfilling.

John A. Colwell, M.D., Ph.D.
President
American Diabetes Association
1987–1988

Acknowledgments

We would like to thank our many expert reviewers for their time and expertise, including Frank Vinicor, M.D.; Pasquale J. Palumbo, M.D.; Carlos Abraira, M.D.; Peter A. Lodewick, M.D.; Louise E. Goggans, D.M.Sc., R.D.; Condit Steil, Pharm.D.; Kathleen Wishner, Ph.D., M.D.; Belinda P. Childs, R.N., M.S.N.; Rena R. Wing, Ph.D.; and Larry C. Deeb, M.D. Thanks are also extended to Michael Brownlee, M.D.; and John Gwynne, M.D., co-chairs of the Council on Complications, and Edward Horton, M.D., Chairman of the Council on Exercise.

This book was revised and produced with contributions from the staff of the American Diabetes Association National Center, including Craig Steinburg, Janice T. Radak, Robin Scott, Susan H. Lau, Caroline Stevens, John C. Warren, and Christine B. Welch.

Table of Contents

Table of Contents

ADA

(American Diabetes Association)

The letters stand for the American Diabetes Association, publisher of this book, *Diabetes A to Z*. The Association is the nation's largest voluntary health organization dedicated to improving the well-being of all people with diabetes and their families. Equally important is our unceasing support for research to find a preventive and cure for this chronic disease that affects some 14 million Americans.

Membership in the American Diabetes Association puts you in contact with a network of more than 270,000 caring people throughout the United States. Our more than 800 local affiliates and chapters offer support groups, educational programs, counseling, and other special services. Membership also brings 12 issues of our lively patient magazine, *Diabetes Forecast*.

The Association also distributes a free quarterly newsletter with practical advice and helpful hints on living with diabetes. Information on Association membership and programs is available through your local affiliate (listed in the white pages of the phone book), or contact:

American Diabetes Association®, Inc.
Diabetes Information Service Center
1660 Duke Street
Alexandria, VA 22314
Tel: 800-232-3472

adolescence

(add-oh-LES-sens)

Is there anyone who can honestly say adolescence was easy for them? The rapid changes that happen during those years—from puberty to full physical and social maturity—can make it difficult and trying for the youngster and parent as well. It is a time when self-images are fragile, peer acceptance is essential, and rebellion against authority is common.

Diabetes doesn't make adolescence any easier. For one, teenagers don't want to be perceived as different, and those with diabetes may not practice good control in an effort to be like everyone else. Such things as taking injections, pricking fingers for blood tests, eating set amounts of food at set times, and dealing with fluctuating blood sugars do not always fit in with a young person's activities and might be ignored.

Such behavior may shock and worry parents, who may try to force proper diabetes control on their youngster. While the gesture may be admirable, it may backfire. Many teens rebel against their diabetes as a show of independence, and tightening control over a teen may cause renewed rebellion.

The teen's attempt to grow up and become more independent is natural and is, in fact, an important step to becoming a mature adult. With patience and willingness to listen to the child's concerns, parents can often help the teen mature while maintaining acceptable levels of diabetes care along the way. To help the child become more independent with respect to diabetes, parents should allow the teen to make his or her own decisions about proper diabetes care. Parents need to relinquish control gradually by allowing the teen to take responsibility—when ready—in such things as urine and blood testing, and insulin adjustments. Of course, mistakes will be made but the youngster will learn from them and may eventually manage diabetes better because of it.

However, if your adolescent son or daughter persists in avoiding self-care—or if other problems seem to be getting out of hand—counseling is an option worth exploring. Counseling for the entire family is often very useful in working on the problems of adolescence, since many of the problems that arise involve not just the adolescent but the interactions of the family as a whole. A doctor or other concerned health professionals may be able to direct you to an experienced counselor. Your local American Diabetes Association chapter or affiliate may have names of counselors with a particular interest in diabetes.

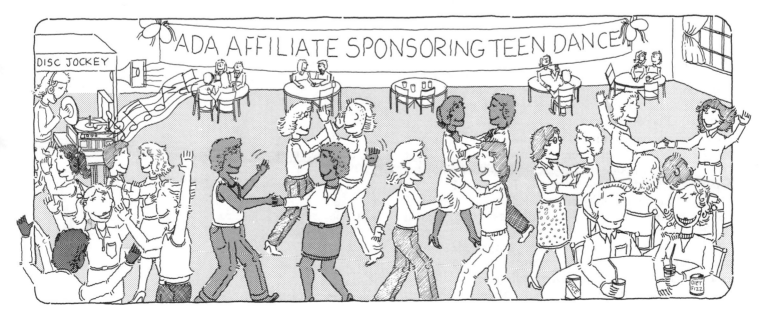

aerobics

Some affiliates also offer social groups and projects for teens. Participating in these programs can help adolescents feel as if they belong and help them feel good about themselves. Being happy with themselves was something many young adults say made all the difference in their lives. When they learned to like themselves—diabetes and all—they somehow found the strength to stick more closely to their diabetes control program.

aerobics

(air-OH-biks)

See Exercise

aging

(AGE-eeng)

They call them the golden years—from age 65 on—and for most of us, they can be if we overcome some of the obstacles of old age. While health problems are a major concern, they don't have to rule a person's life. As people who keep their diabetes in control know, the secret is to prevent problems or at least catch them before they get worse.

High blood pressure, arthritis, atherosclerosis (hardening of the arteries, see Atherosclerosis), eye problems, and mobility problems are all complications that should be of concern to the entire older population and not just individuals with diabetes. These problems may not become major ones if the proper care is taken to prevent them. Regular checkups with your doctor are a step in the right direction.

For the person who has not had diabetes, some of the symptoms—or the disease itself—could appear in later life. The ability to keep blood sugars in the non-diabetic range after meals (your glucose tolerance) declines a bit as people grow older. This process usually begins when a person is in his/her 30s. Once a person is over 60, his or her blood-glucose levels after meals are likely to rise to levels that are above normal but not in a range that we call diabetes. Today, we say these individuals have *impaired glucose tolerance* (IGT). While some studies show that IGT may be a normal sign of aging, other studies show that IGT is the first step on the road to developing diabetes. That's why we encourage all people with IGT to have yearly check-ups with their doctors. (See Impaired Glucose Tolerance.)

And we encourage all older people to continue eating balanced meals—as with young people with diabetes, proper nutrition is all important. The meal plans devised by the American Diabetes Association (see Exchange Lists) are good guidelines for healthy eating, whether you have diabetes or not. Also, it is a good idea to discuss *your* individual nutritional needs with your doctor or dietitian.

OK, you have taken care of your physical needs—what's next? Start living! Just because you are a little older doesn't mean you have to sit home in that overstuffed chair you have grown fond of over the years. In fact, if you do, you may just get bored with life or worse, become terribly depressed.

You may want to take part in community activities. Many people have become involved in volunteer work. You probably carry with you mounds of experience that others would find valuable. If you would like to volunteer, check the newspapers for "volunteers wanted" ads. Your local church, library, or town hall may be able to steer you in the right direction.

You could pursue interests you never were able to do because of time restraints (like learning to play the piano, or golf or sew). If you are lonely, get out and meet people. Agencies such as the "Y," local churches and synagogues, senior citizens' clubs, community centers, and parks departments often have a variety of activities and information at low or no cost.

alcohol

(AL-co-HALL)

While most people can enjoy moderate drinking without much worry to their health, people with diabetes need to give more thought to their use of alcohol. For one, alcohol can lower blood glucose levels by impairing the manufacture, storage, and release of glucose by your liver. Drinking alcohol on an empty stomach should always be avoided—such a practice could lower your blood glucose level enough to cause hypoglycemia, if you take insulin or oral antihypoglycemic agents (see Oral Agents). Alcohol can also raise blood sugar, especially in people whose diabetes is poorly controlled.

Another thing to consider is that alcohol can impair a person's judgment. A person who has had a number of drinks may forget to take an injection or may forget to eat, or may even snack excessively on party food. Worse, if a person who has been drinking experiences hypoglycemia, people at the party may dismiss it as effects from alcohol and not treat the hypoglycemic reaction. Also, if you take oral medication

in the spirits

Beverage	Serving Size	Approx. Cal.	Number of Exchanges
Distilled Spirits (86 proof)	1½ oz.	107	2½ Fats
Dry Table Wine (12% alcohol)	3 oz.	68	1½ Fats
Wine Cooler (6% alcohol)	12 oz.	196	3 Fats, 1 Bread
Regular Beer (4.5% alcohol)	12 oz.	151	3½ Fats, or 2 Fats, 1 Bread
"Light" Beer (3.5% alcohol)	12 oz.	97	2 Fats

to treat your diabetes, alcohol may block the medication's ability to work properly and may make you feel sick.

So, does all this mean a person with diabetes can't drink? Not necessarily. What it does mean is that alcohol, like all aspects of diabetes care, should be approached sensibly. Thus, it might do you well to heed the following advice:

■ If you choose to drink you should first check with your physician to see how much alcohol, if any, is safe for you and how you can fit it into your diet. Although alcohol is made from carbohydrates, it is digested like a fat in the body and is classified as a Fat Exchange (see chart).

■ Always eat something when you drink. Alcohol can lower blood glucose, and eating will help prevent hypoglycemic reactions. Skipping or delaying a meal is the main cause of hypoglycemia.

■ Hold a drink for a long time, and take tiny sips. That way you can avoid frequent refills.

■ Avoid sweet wines, liqueurs, and sweetened mixers. If you need a mixer, use a sugar-free soft drink, club soda, seltzer, or water. Light beer is a better choice than regular beer because it has less alcohol and fewer carbohydrates.

■ If you are reading this article with extreme eagerness, ask yourself why. If being able to drink is an important priority to you, you might be inclined toward chronic, habitual drinking. It is especially important for a person with diabetes to seek help when drinking becomes a problem. According to the National Council on Alcoholism, the signs of problem drinking include: (1) an inability to control how much you drink; (2) feeling guilty about your drinking, regretting things you did or said while drinking; (3) looking forward to drinking; and (4) consuming an average of 14 drinks per week.

If any of these signs seem familiar, consult your doctor. You can also contact Alcoholics Anonymous or the local affiliate of the National Council on Alcoholism.

■ If you decide not to drink, there are lots of alternatives. You don't have to apologize for not drinking. Rather, gracefully ask for a nonalcoholic alternative. Mineral, spring, or sparkling, natural water are options. Or choose your favorite diet soda.

American Diabetes Association

(American DI-a-BEET-eez Association)

The world's leading voluntary health agency concerned with finding a cure for diabetes, as well as treating individuals with the disease (see ADA).

amputation

(AM-pew-TAY-shun)

Amputation is not the most pleasant topic to discuss. But did you know that diabetes is responsible for most amputations? (Amputation is the surgical removal of a toe, part of a foot, a hand, or even part of an arm or leg.) Because amputation is a reality for some people with diabetes, understanding the operation and the rehabilitation that is available will help, should this happen to you.

One of the reasons people with diabetes are more at risk for amputations is because they are more vulnerable to foot problems. Two foot problems that may eventually lead to amputation, if not properly controlled, are neuropathy (nerve damage—see Neuropathy) and circulatory problems (which can limit or block blood flow). Sometimes amputation is necessary to correct serious, poor circulation problems.

Neuropathy is serious because it can limit your ability to feel pain. You may step on a nail or get a blister or burn on your foot without knowing it. If you don't treat the damage, your foot could get infected (see Foot Care). Under normal conditions, your body would attack the infection with white blood cells. But if you are also having circulatory problems, the blood can't get to where it is needed and heal the infection. If the damaged area does not heal, the infection could spread and gangrene could set in (see Gangrene). If this happens, amputation may be necessary to stop the infection from spreading.

The amount that has to be amputated is determined by evaluating the circulation in the leg and calculating the place farthest down the leg or foot that has a chance of healing. Sometimes vascular surgery is an alternative to amputation. A vascular surgeon may be able to remove a blood-vessel blockage to restore circulation.

Physical therapy begins several days after surgery and includes working on parallel bars, a walker, and crutches to regain balance. Therapy also helps a person learn how to fall safely and how to get up.

When part of the leg is removed, an artificial limb (prosthesis) is fitted once the leg has healed. When part of the foot is amputated, a prosthesis is made to fill out a shoe and protect the remaining part of the foot. Physical therapy also helps a person learn how to walk with the new limb.

Of course, it's better to try to keep the real thing. So you will want to do what you can to prevent an amputation. Many experts believe that amputations can be prevented through proper self-care, including keeping your diabetes in control, examining your feet daily, and having regular checkups with your doctor. Taking the proper precautions may make all the difference.

anger

(ANG-ger)

You secrete more adrenalin. Your heart starts to beat faster. Your body releases more sugar. The pupils in your eyes dilate. Your blood pressure rises— and pow!—your temper flies out of control.

Anger is one of those things we all experience occasionally and it is not unusual for a person to become angry once they have been diagnosed with diabetes. First, there is the coping with the diagnosis and then with the changes in lifestyle. Later, you may feel angry when you are treated differently

animals

in public—when people focus on the disease and overlook the whole person. Being accused of cheating on diabetes care can be another cause for anger.

Whatever the reason, we all need to work at managing angry feelings and using them constructively. Here are a few suggestions:

■ Recognize that your feelings are normal. It is natural to feel angry when something negative happens to you. Acknowledging your anger is the first step to adjustment.

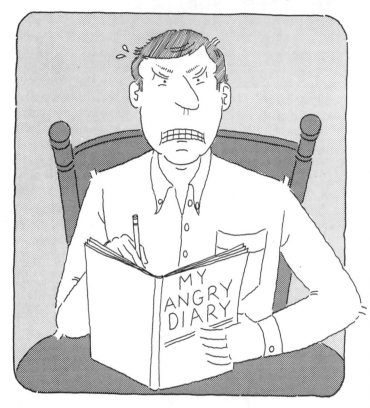

■ Identify the sources of your anger and substitute productive ways to deal with your anger. You may want to keep a diary of those things that make you angry. Later, sit down with your entries and decide how you will handle a similar situation in the future.

If you sense you are becoming angry try some of these techniques to calm yourself:

■ Talk more slowly. It is difficult to yell slowly.
■ Breath longer and more deeply.
■ If you are standing, sit down. Sitting down helps settle your anger and makes you more comfortable.
■ Get yourself a drink of water. This will literally help cool you off.

animals

(ANN-i-MALLS)

What went through the mind of the first recipient of insulin? That's hard to say, but what is known is that as soon as she started feeling better, she stood up and wagged her tail. For almost a century, researchers have been enlisting animals in the search for answers to the puzzles of diabetes.

The animals that are now helping diabetes researchers would make up a rather odd-looking collection. They include dogs, mice, hamsters, monkeys, rats, and even a special breed of pig called Yucatan miniature swine. Without them, diabetes research would proceed at a snail's pace.

Diabetes in animals is often used as a model, or representation, of diabetes as it occurs in humans. Different kinds of animals develop different kinds of diabetes. The Egyptian sand rat, for example, sometimes develops a form of diabetes—caused by a long bout of overeating—that resembles human non-insulin-dependent (type II) diabetes.

By contrast, the spontaneously diabetic BioBreeding (BB) rat develops a form of insulin-dependent (type I) diabetes with many of the same symptoms—such as extreme thirst—that occur in people. Some Yucatan miniature swine even seem to mimic human gestational diabetes—they only become diabetic during pregnancy.

To paraphrase Shakespeare, some animals are born with diabetes, while others have diabetes thrust upon them. Marjorie, the dog on the receiving end of Banting and Best's first insulin injection, acquired diabetes through removal of her pancreas (see History of Diabetes). Nowadays, researchers inject animals with chemicals that destroy the insulin-producing beta cells. Others, however, are selectively bred because they have a genetic tendency toward diabetes.

Because scientists learn a great deal from these studies, the American Diabetes Association supports responsible and humane care and use of laboratory animals in research. The Association also encourages the development and use of alternatives to live animals when possible.

While using animals provides valuable answers to the mysteries of diabetes, scientists do have to be cautious in making assumptions about human diabetes on the basis of results seen in animals. This is because they are not identical to human beings, and the causes and treatments of their diabetes might be different from those for people.

Diabetes in animals is not just a product of laboratory testing, however. Sometimes the family pet—be it dog, cat, or parrot—develops the well-known symptoms, including thirst, hunger, and weight loss. The key to controlling diabetes in a pet is the same as that for a person—a consistent balance of insulin, food, and exercise.

Insulin doses for dogs and cats vary from 1 to 40 units a day. Birds generally require a fraction of a unit. Periodic urine tests for sugar and ketones will help the owner make sure that the diabetes is staying under reasonable control.

Diabetes control is an added responsibility for a pet owner, but with good control there is no reason why your pet can't live a long and happy life. After all that animals have done for us, caring for them is the least we can do!

anorexia

(ANN-or-X-see-ah)

Anorexia means not having an appetite for food. Many people experience short periods of anorexia during their lifetimes. *Anorexia nervosa* is an extreme, unusual, but serious psychological problem that most often occurs in young women. Individuals suffering from anorexia nervosa refuse to maintain a normal, healthy body weight. Even though they are grossly underweight, they see themselves as being overweight. Basically, they are scared of gaining weight.

People suffering from anorexia nervosa need medical and psychological help. This disorder is extremely dangerous, especially for the person with diabetes. Proper diabetes control is achieved by balancing food and insulin. For adolescents, this balance is necessary to ensure proper growth and development. A dose of insulin combined with too little food can result in low blood sugar (see Hypoglycemia) and cause an insulin reaction.

If you are suffering from anorexia nervosa, whether you have diabetes or not, get medical help immediately. With the proper medical and psychological help, you can overcome this problem.

A₁C

(a-one-see)

See Glycosylated Hemoglobin

atherosclerosis

(ATH-er-o-skluh-row-sis)

It's no coincidence that large highways are often referred to as "major arteries." In many ways, your circulatory system is just like a system of roadways. In both systems, the major arteries are used to transport large amounts of important products (such as food and fuel on the roads, oxygen and nutrients through the blood vessels) across large distances. Then they branch off into smaller and smaller "side streets" that make "local deliveries" possible.

Atherosclerosis, simply put, is closing the traffic lanes and causing traffic congestion. It comes about when excess cholesterol, calcium, and connective tissue build up on the inner wall of a large blood vessel and restrict the flow of blood. People with diabetes run a higher risk than others of developing atherosclerosis. Atherosclerosis is the major cause of heart disease and occurs two to four times more often in people with diabetes. But there are steps everyone can take to help keep "traffic" moving.

Atherosclerosis belongs to a class of blood-vessel disorders called *macroangiopathies*. This means that it strikes the larger blood vessels, such as those in the legs, thighs, neck, and heart. Atherosclerosis is a common cause of large blood-vessel disease, often referred to as macrovascular complications. It especially affects the major arteries that carry blood to the heart, head, and legs. Atherosclerosis causes the blood vessel walls to become thick and rigid (lose their elasticity) and the opening in the artery to become narrow. Also, the inner lining of the walls becomes caked with calcium and fatlike patches.

What are the signs of atherosclerosis? That depends in part on where in the body it is occurring. But one general symptom is pain. Often, pain will occur only while the part of the body nourished by the narrowed vessel is more active than usual. If the heart, for example, is beating harder because of exercise (such as walking up stairs) or stress, and if it needs more oxygen and nutrients than the arteries feeding it can provide, the result is often a pain known as *angina*. The same thing can happen in the legs and feet: often a person with atherosclerosis in the legs will feel pain while walking but not while standing or sitting. (This is called *intermittent claudication*.)

In fact, the legs and feet are where atherosclerosis most often strikes people with diabetes. Other signs of atherosclerosis in the legs include cold feet, loss of hair on the feet, and redness when the feet are allowed to dangle (for instance, when you are sitting on a table and allow your feet to hang over the edge). The redness in your feet is a sign that, because of poor circulation, the blood cannot make its way back out of the foot.

If you experience any such signs, see your physician. Doctors have a variety of tests available to them to find out if you have atherosclerosis and to pinpoint where it is occurring. Treatment may include stricter meal planning or medication, but sometimes the only way to correct a blockage is through surgery.

What are the steps a person can take to prevent atherosclerosis?

■ Don't smoke. People who smoke run a far higher risk of atherosclerosis than nonsmokers.

■ Reduce calories if you are overweight. Slimming down to your ideal weight should be your top priority for fighting atherosclerosis. Cut down on both excess fat (butter, meat fat) and concentrated sugar.

■ Cut cholesterol. Keeping your cholesterol intake to less than 300 milligrams per day is a good practice. The "typical" American diet contains 400 to 500 milligrams of cholesterol per day. One step toward lowering cholesterol is to substitute saturated fats (animal fats) with polyunsaturated fats (vegetable fats) in your diet. This is because saturated fats tend to increase the levels of cholesterol in the blood. It is also a good idea to reduce your intake of foods that actually contain cholesterol (such as eggs, red meats, and organ meats, such as liver).

■ Control high blood pressure. Exercising regularly, reducing salt in the diet, and taking prescribed medications will help achieve this.

babies

(BAY-bees)

Cute, cuddly, smart, loving, friendly, bright, happy—sound like someone you know? We all tend to think our babies are exceptional, and you know something, we're right. Because they are so special, they deserve the best possible

bag lunches

care we can give them. For the parent who has an infant with diabetes, it may mean more work, but proper diabetes care will help junior develop into a healthy, active child.

First, you need to have a diabetes specialist and other members of your diabetes care team teach you how to adjust insulin and diet so your infant will grow and develop normally. Your baby will need food to balance insulin. This can be a difficult task since there will be times when your infant will refuse to eat. When this happens offer your baby something else. If your baby is still on liquids, offer a variety of fluids. If solids have been introduced, alternate between solids and fluids. If that doesn't work, wait a few minutes and try again.

Forcing the little darling to eat may only lead to more frustration and stress—both for you and the child. More than likely, this fussiness is part of normal development and will pass. You may have to settle for feeding your baby only the food he or she likes for a time. For the child with diabetes, that is a better alternative than no food at all.

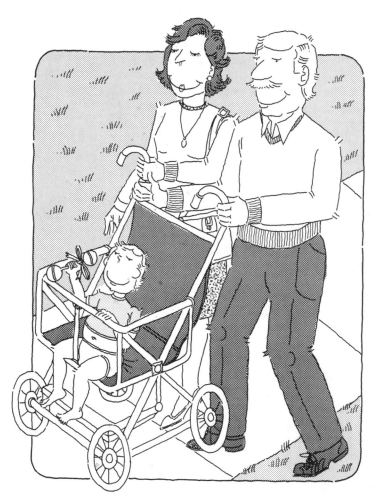

Besides being concerned about your baby's eating habits, you may worry about insulin reactions. You may worry because your baby cannot tell you when he or she feels that a reaction may be coming on. Don't worry, just look for signs: sweating, pallor (paleness), irritability, a sudden change in personality (suddenly stops playing), lethargy (tiredness), shaking, restlessness during the night, cyanosis (bluish color around the lips), or dilated pupils.

Blood testing should be done to determine if your baby's blood-sugar level is low. All parents of infants with diabetes should know how to test blood sugar. Taking a blood sample from the heels, toes, or earlobes may be a good alternative to tiny fingers. (However, if your child is walking, you may want to avoid pricking the feet to avoid infections.) You can test for urine sugar by gently pressing a urine test strip on a wet diaper to get a reading. It is *essential* that you test your baby's urine for ketones.

If your baby's blood glucose is low, give him or her some form of sugar. (Follow your doctor's advice when to treat.) You can give your baby a sugary drink such as orange juice, sugar water, or sugar-sweetened Kool-Aid. Be sure to follow the sugar with a long-acting protein or complex carbohydrate, such as formula or milk. If your infant is on solids, you can substitute cereal, vegetables, or meat for the milk. If your baby will not eat or is not improving, give a glucagon injection and call your physician for further advice. (Glucagon is a hormone that raises blood sugar. See Glucagon.) Be sure to have your diabetes specialist give you guidelines on glucagon injections.

Worrying about your child is normal, whether your baby has diabetes or not. Sharing the responsibility with your spouse, parents, or a trusted friend will help you cope with your baby's diabetes. Also, don't forget to take advantage of the support members of a health-care team (physicians, educators, social service people) if these resources are available.

bag lunches
(BAG LUNCH-es)

Bringing your own lunch has its advantages: The food is made just the way you like it in just the right amount; it's there when you want it, no waiting for service; and it's economical—no restaurant taxes to pay, and no tips. Speaking of tips:

■ Keep bread from becoming soggy from moist fillings by spreading it with a thin layer of margarine—or try ricotta cheese or mayonnaise. Easy on the mayo, though, and remember it can go bad in the heat.

■ Freeze enough sandwiches for a week. But don't add mayonnaise or salad dressing until the day you use the sandwich; these spreads separate when they are frozen.

■ To keep food cool, wrap a can of frozen juice in a plastic bag and pack it with your lunch.

■ Separately package "wet" foods, such as tomatoes, pickles, and lettuce.

■ Remember that leftovers make great lunches.

■ Include a variety of textures and tastes to keep the meal interesting. Mix tart and sweet, soft and crunchy foods. Vary the breads, too. Have pumpernickel one day, whole wheat or French bread the next.

■ Consider alternatives to sandwiches: hearty soups, stews, inventive salads, or cheese and bread with fresh fruit for dessert.

beach

(BEECH)

Diabetes does not have to interfere with your summer fun, but before you roll out the beach blanket, here are a few things to keep in mind:

■ Barefoot is not the way to go. Broken glass, bottle caps, and sea shells all lurk just beneath that smooth sand, waiting to set your feet on the royal road to infection. What's more, sand can be hot: if you have neuropathy you may not realize your feet are being burned.

■ If you are taking your insulin to the seashore, consider stashing it in the cooler to keep it from overheating. Take it out a short time before use to let it warm to a comfortable temperature.

■ The warm weather encourages some people to lie down and relax, while it spurs others to dive into the water or join in a game of touch football. Changing your activity levels in either direction can require modification of your eating patterns and insulin dose (for the insulin user).

■ If you take insulin, take a buddy along for that plunge into the pool or the sea. The extra activity of swimming can help lower your blood-glucose level, which is fine, unless it leads to an insulin reaction. In that case, you'll want to be on solid ground.

■ Whether you are lying down or running around, the hot weather at the beach means more sweating, leading to a loss of body fluid. If your diabetes is not well controlled, you may be slightly dehydrated already, and the extra water loss won't help. So drink more fluids during warm weather, and if possible have your own supply at the beach.

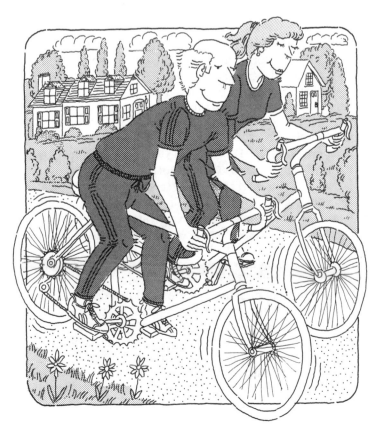

■ A burn is a burn—whether caused by fire or the sun. And sunburn, like other injuries, can lead to infection. Use a sunscreen that blocks the ultraviolet rays of the sun (the rays that burn). But don't just rely on sunscreens—wear a hat or use an umbrella when you can.

bicycling

(BYE-sik-clean)

When you think of exercising, does the word "fun" come to mind? If not, maybe you aren't thinking about bicycling. Not only is cycling fun, it is one of the safest aerobic exercises around.

Cycling improves cardiovascular fitness by conditioning your heart, lungs, and circulatory system without giving your feet, ankles, and knees the pounding other exercises do. If you have type I diabetes, regular bicycling may help improve your body's sensitivity to insulin. If you have type II diabetes, regular aerobic exercise can help you lose weight and possibly reduce your need for medication.

Cycling easily adapts to your fitness level and interests. If you're looking for recreation and relaxation, try a leisurely ride on a local bike path or through the quiet streets in your neighborhood. Or, put your bike to work for you; use it to commute to and from work or the store.

Now that we've got you excited about cycling, let's talk about your wheels. If you have a bike that has been out of commission, you'll want to take it to a bike shop for a tune-up. If you're in the market for a new bike, find one that is the proper size for you. It is important that you be able to straddle the bike and stand flat-footed on the ground with an inch or two of clearance above the top tube.

Next, you'll want to be sure your seat height is adjusted properly. To check your seat-height adjustment, put one pedal down in its lowest position. Place the ball of your foot on the pedal. If your seat is adjusted right, your knee will be slightly bent in this position.

Now that you have chosen your bicycle, the next piece of equipment you should buy is a helmet. Wherever you ride—around your neighborhood, through city streets, or across country—wear a helmet. While we are on the subject of safety, remember to take some precautions. If you take insulin, check your blood-glucose level before setting out for a ride. If you're above 250 mg/dl and test positive for ketones, postpone your ride until you have your diabetes under better control.

Be sure to carry a quick-acting carbohydrate (sugar packet, hard candy, glucose gel) in case of an insulin reaction. Stop and treat a reaction at once; do not try to make it home.

Since cycling primarily uses your leg muscles, your doctor may advise you to inject in some site other than the thigh before riding. Injecting near an exercising muscle may help your insulin to be absorbed faster. Don't take your insulin injections in the thigh or hip before cycling, because the insulin absorption will be increased. Now, check your tires and brakes, adjust your seat, fasten your helmet, and pedal on. Oh yes, try to remember you're exercising.

binges

(BIN-jez)

We all like to eat and most of us indulge from time to time. But for some, overeating to the point of gluttony is like an addiction. Binging can be a serious problem and difficult to control.

Binging can be extremely harmful to your health, especially if you have diabetes. Good diabetes control requires that you follow a sensible meal plan.

(If you binge and then use laxatives, water pills or diuretics, or vomiting to get rid of the food, you have a serious problem. See Bulimia.)

To stop binge eating, you first need the determination to stop. You may need to seek professional advice (such as a doctor or a therapist) to help you avoid taking that "one little bite" that leads to all the rest. In addition, you may benefit from continued support from family, friends, and self-help groups (such as Weight Watchers or Overeaters Anonymous). Check your phone book.

Here are approaches that have helped some people to control binge eating:

■ Take inventory. List the ways your binges limit your life and make you unhappy. Also, to become aware of "high-risk" situations and the things that trigger your binges, keep track of the food you eat—what, when, where—for a week. Then list your ideas for avoiding or coping with the situations and triggers. For instance, if you tend to binge when you are angry, consider expressing the anger directly or writing it out.

■ Keep binge foods out of the house...Don't buy them yourself, and ask your family to cooperate.

■ Don't skip meals...You'll get too hungry to control yourself. And resolve to eat *only* at the table—never standing up or right out of the container.

■ Set up a support system of people you can call when the cravings begin to overpower you.

■ Stop and think... Before you grab the food, ask yourself, "Am I really hungry?" Visualize how you will feel after the binge. Is the momentary gratification worth the blood-sugar jolt, the cramps, the nausea, and the never-ending visits to the bathroom, not to mention the guilt and the worry about complications?

■ Put it off... Tell yourself you can have the food—but *later*. Often the craving will pass.

■ Do something...anything. Take a walk. Draw a bath. Jog. Wash the car. Have a list of activities you enjoy ready in advance.

■ Be prepared... If you *must* have *something*, try to make it one portion of a food you enjoy, but one that won't lead to an uncontrolled eating spree. Don't wolf it down. Eat slowly, tasting and savoring every bite so you'll feel satisfied. Try popcorn. Three full cups cooked (no oil) amounts to only 70 calories (1 Starch/Bread Exchange).

■ Be on your own side... For one woman who finally gained control over binging, the turning point came when she realized that if someone else in her family were the one with diabetes, she would do everything to see that person had the proper diet.

■ Change your thinking about food... Instead of bemoaning the foods you cannot eat, think about the foods you can eat. Find permissible foods (perhaps a favorite fruit) that will feel like a treat whenever you have it. If you hate your meal plan or always feel hungry, talk to your dietitian about ways to make permissible foods more satisfying.

■ See your doctor... Perpetual hunger is sometimes a sign that your diabetes treatment plan needs changes.

■ Don't be a perfectionist... For many people, the urge to binge never goes away completely. To think you will never slip is unrealistic and sets you up for failure. If you slip up, do not give up. Forgive yourself and start over.

birth control

(BERTH con-TROL)

When it comes to birth control, couples have several options. There is the condom, the pill, intrauterine devices (IUDs), the diaphragm, spermicidal foams, vasectomy, tubal ligation, and, uh, even abstinence. If that last one is *not* an option for you, read on.

Of course, people who use birth control want something that has a high success rate ("failure," when it comes to birth control, is another way of saying "pregnancy"). People with diabetes also want to use something that will not affect their diabetes control. According to experts, you can use whatever form of birth control *you* prefer—as long as you are aware of special precautions.

One popular method of birth control for women is the pill. There are two basic types: the combination pill, which contains estrogen and progestogens (sex hormones), and the progestogen-only pill. Doctors favor the combination pill because it is slightly more effective: 99 percent versus 98 percent. The progestogen-only pill can also cause irregular bleeding and weight gain.

If you have insulin-dependent (type I) diabetes, the combined pill can interfere with diabetes control. So, if you go on the pill, you may have to increase the amount of insulin you inject.

In women with type I diabetes, the short-term risks (a year or two) are slight, but scientists are not certain about the risks of using the pill for longer periods of time. If you develop high blood pressure while taking the pill, this could increase the risk that retinopathy or kidney disease will progress. Because of this, you need to know if you have any complications before you start using birth control pills.

Condoms are another form of birth control you may want to consider. As with all forms of birth control, the condom is not 100 percent effective. While condoms do present a margin of error, some types of condoms may help prevent the transmission of sexual diseases, such as herpes and acquired immune deficiency syndrome (AIDS). (Unfortunately, there is no guarantee that condoms will prevent the transmission of AIDS. Transmission can occur through the pores of some condoms. Also, breakage of a condom does sometimes occur, eliminating protection from AIDS and pregnancy as well.)

IUDs are fitted inside a woman's uterus by a doctor. Many IUDs were taken off the market because they were suspected to cause pelvic infections in those women who used them. Because they are linked with infections, IUDs generally are not recommended for women who have diabetes. Discuss with your doctor any benefits or risks involved to see if using an IUD is a good choice for you.

Another method of birth control for women is the diaphragm. This is a dome-shaped rubber cup that is inserted in the vagina just before intercourse. For best results, you should use a spermicide (sperm-killing gel) with it. The diaphragm can be an effective means of birth control as long as it is used properly. A diaphragm's effectiveness depends on whether it is fitted and inserted properly. It isn't harmful, but if your doctor says it may not be reliable for you, try something else.

Some couples opt for tubal ligation or a vasectomy. Both of these require surgery, but if you think you may want children some day, it is important to remember neither of these techniques is reversible with any degree of certainty. If you have such a procedure, be sure the doctor in charge is aware of your diabetes and pays special attention to diabetes control before, during, and after the procedure.

Whatever method of birth control you decide to use, remember that both partners share the responsibility for birth control.

blood glucose
(BLUD GLOO-kose)

Having diabetes means learning all about blood glucose. But what exactly is glucose? Glucose is a simple form of sugar (we interchange the terms blood sugar and blood glucose—they mean the same thing). It is produced when the foods you eat, particularly carbohydrates, are broken down into simple nutrients in your digestive system. Glucose is the main fuel that powers people, and it is as necessary to us as gasoline is to cars.

Your body's cells "burn" glucose to get the energy your body needs to perform daily tasks. The glucose travels to the cells through the blood.

When the body is functioning as it should, the level of glucose in the blood is kept within a very narrow range—around 70 to 120 mg/dl before meals and no higher than 140 to 160 mg/dl several hours after meals (mg/dl means "milligrams of glucose per deciliter of blood"). If blood sugar is on the rise, as it is after a meal, the nondiabetic body keeps it within this range by secreting insulin. Insulin is the hormone (or key) that "unlocks" the body's cells to allow glucose to enter. The sugar enters the cells, and the blood glucose level goes down. If there is more glucose than the body cells need at the moment, the sugar is stored in the cells of the liver or converted to fat.

But in diabetes, something goes wrong with the insulin—it is either in short supply or is not being used properly by the cells. When this happens, glucose cannot get into the cells (there is no "key" to open the "lock" to let glucose in).

Glucose then starts accumulating in the blood. Eventually, excess glucose is filtered out of the blood and "spills over" into the urine. This is why people with uncontrolled diabetes have large amounts of sugar in their urine.

It's thought that high levels of blood glucose contribute to many long-term complications of diabetes, including retinopathy and heart and kidney disease. Fortunately, blood glucose can often be kept in or near the normal range by proper balancing of insulin, diet, and exercise. Advances such as portable blood glucose monitors (see Self-monitoring) have made diabetes more manageable. The coming years promise more ways to make sure a person's blood is never any sweeter than it should be.

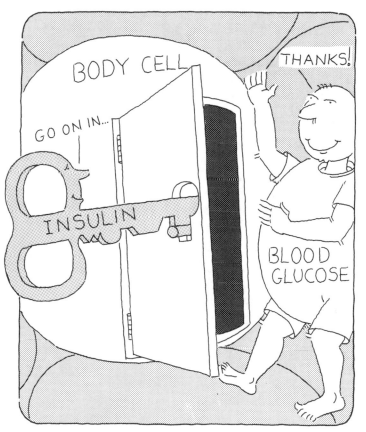

blood tests
(BLUD TESTS)

To keep your diabetes in control, you and your doctor need to know your blood glucose level. The best way to find this out is through blood tests that provide an accurate reading of how much glucose is in your blood.

In fact, there are many blood tests that your doctor may perform before ever diagnosing diabetes. These can include the oral glucose tolerance test, fasting blood glucose tests and random blood glucose tests. But these relate almost exclusively to diagnosis. There are simple blood tests that *you* can do to help control your diabetes. . .and that's what we'll discuss here.

bulimia

Blood-glucose tests are more accurate than urine-glucose tests because they show you the exact amount of glucose in your blood at the time of the test. Urine tests are faulty because they can only give you an estimate of the level of glucose actually present in your blood over a period of time. This is especially true if you have not emptied your bladder for a while. If this is the case, the test will give you results of what the blood-sugar level was several hours before the test rather than what it is when you take the test. Urine tests also cannot tell you when you have low blood sugar. When a urine test is negative, your blood sugar can be anywhere from below 60 mg to almost 200 mg. (That's because sugar doesn't pass from the blood to the urine until the sugar tops about 180 mg.) And when a urine test is positive for sugar, your blood glucose could be upwards of 700 mg! So, if you're looking for accuracy, blood tests are your best bet.

With the aid of a portable glucose monitor or visual strips, you can check your blood-glucose levels daily. The American Diabetes Association recommends that you test your own blood (called self-monitoring) if you use insulin, are pregnant, are prone to severe ketosis or severe hypoglycemia (low blood sugar), or have a high renal threshold (the point at which glucose spills over into the urine).

If you test regularly and record the results, you and your doctor can accurately follow the course of your diabetes. The blood tests will be a great educator. They will show you how stress, foods (protein, complex carbohydrates, and sugar), exercise, and medicine affect your blood sugar. This will help you and your physician know how to alter your meal plan and activity level to bring your glucose level as close to normal as possible. Keeping control of your diabetes may mean delaying or preventing the complications of diabetes. And that translates into a healthier, happier life! (See also Glycosylated Hemoglobin and Self-Monitoring.)

bulimia
(byoo-leem-EE-ah)

In our section on "Binges," we discussed the problems of overeating. In this section, we want to talk about a more serious form of binging called bulimia nervosa.

The individual with bulimia typically binges (eats large amounts of food) and then follows with purging (by vomiting or the use of laxatives or water pills/diuretics) and rigid dieting. People suffering from bulimia are overly concerned with the shape and weight of their bodies. Bulimia seems to occur most often in young women—usually in their teens, twenties, and thirties.

Binging and then purging is extremely dangerous to anyone's health. Regular vomiting can cause such serious problems as damage to the liver, kidneys, esophagus, and teeth. Besides vomiting, many individuals with bulimia will take large doses of laxatives or diuretics to prevent them from gaining weight. Abuse of laxatives and diuretics can ruin the normal functioning of the intestinal system. Purging can lead to a loss of potassium, and for people with diabetes, this can play havoc with an already disturbed metabolism. Add this to poor diabetes control, and you could push yourself into a diabetic coma.

If you suffer from bulimia, don't put off getting medical and psychological help. Bulimia can be a life-threatening problem that can be cured, and there are professionals who can help you.

calisthenics
(KAL-ahs-THEN-iks)

See Exercise

camps
(KAMPS)

Remember summer camp—canoeing and swimming, singing around the campfire, exploring nature, and making new friends? Well, camps for kids with diabetes are no different.

There are more than 50 accredited camps in the United States—and all are listed in the American Diabetes Associa-

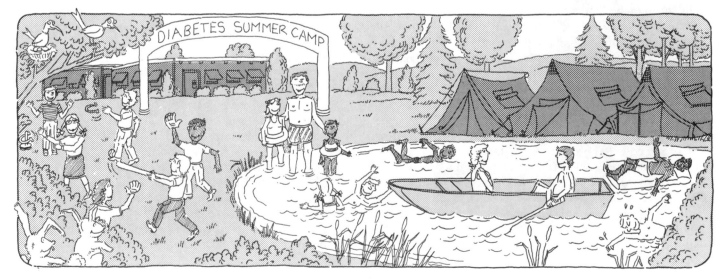

tion's Camp Directory. Each camp offers kids a chance to meet others with diabetes, so they realize they are not alone. The campers have fun while learning more about their diabetes and how to manage it more independently.

Camp is a vacation not only for kids, but for parents too. Camp frees mom and dad of the everyday parenting and diabetes-related responsibilities—and gives them a chance to be alone. Parents also deserve a break.

If you want more information, your local affiliate can direct you to the program nearest you. The American Diabetes Association Camp Directory is revised each year and is made available by March. If you would like a copy, write to:
Camp Directory
American Diabetes Association
National Information Center
1660 Duke Street
Alexandria, VA 22314

carbohydrates
(KAR-bow-HIGH-drates)

There was a time when "carbohydrate" was a dirty word. People thought carbohydrates were more fattening than other foods. Not so. In fact, ounce for ounce, carbohydrates provide half the calories of fat. But any food can be fattening if you eat too much.

There are two types of carbohydrates: *simple* and *complex*. Simple carbohydrates, or sugars, are found in honey, syrup, candy, table sugar, jams and jellies, cakes, pastries, sweetened beverages and desserts. They can be converted quickly into glucose and thus may spell trouble for diabetes control. Complex carbohydrates, or starches, are found in bread, pasta, cereal, rice, beans, and vegetables. These take longer to break down in digestion, and so cause a more gradual increase in blood sugar.

The source of the carbohydrate is important to note. Natural food sources—such as fresh fruits and milk form simple carbohydrates, whole grains and fresh vegetables form complex carbohydrates—are good for getting many of the nutrients you need, such as vitamins, minerals, and fiber. But simple carbohydrates can also be refined (for example, table sugar). In refining, carbohydrates lose much of their nutritional value but retain their calories. These refined sugars should be limited, especially for people with diabetes.

Remember, when working with your meal plan, don't forget to include complex carbohydrates. Besides being full of vitamins and minerals, they also are a great source of energy. Check the American Diabetes Association's *Exchange Lists for Meal Planning* for help in determining how much carbohydrate you can work into your meal plan.

cheating
(CHEE-teeng)

Have you ever caught yourself or been accused of cheating on your diabetes control? Maybe you were walking past a bakery shop, decided that a few extra bread, fruit, and fat exchanges wouldn't be noticed by anyone, and then later you felt guilty. Or maybe you really thought you *were* sticking to your meal plan, but your doctor, after weighing you, accused you of "noncompliance." Whatever the case, no one likes to be accused of "cheating."

Unless you are superhuman, you probably have cheated on your meal plan at one time or another. Occasional "slips" should not cause you to despair or feel guilty. Sticking to your meal plan is a tough challenge; the trick is to meet this challenge positively.

The person who cheats constantly isn't the only one hurt by it. Watching a loved one do something that is not healthy can be painful for friends and family as well. Here are some tips to help you avoid cheating on your diabetes regimen:

■ Learn how to fit the foods you love most into your meal plan. This will let you enjoy your food rather than feel guilty about eating it. The better you understand your meal plan and the Exchange List meal-planning system, the healthier and more flexible your life will be. If you could easily become a cake and ice cream junkie, this approach may not work. But, by knowing how the meal plan system works, you may well be able to fit these foods into special-occasion meal plans. Just don't make every day a special occasion.
■ Keep busy. Boredom is a leading cause of nibbling.
■ Check your blood sugar. Low blood sugar can cause hunger. And if you are hungry, you may eat foods you shouldn't. If low blood sugar occurs frequently, your doctor and dietitian may decide you need to readjust medication or add calories to your diet.
■ Depression, loneliness, anxiety, and other negative emotions may also cause you to eat more than you need. A heart-to-heart talk with a friend or counselor could help.
■ Exercise! It will help get your mind off food, give you a lift, and make you feel fit and in control. Exercise can even help decrease your appetite.

What if someone else accuses you of cheating because you aren't losing weight or your blood or urine tests show high sugar levels? This can be frustrating, especially if you believe that you have been faithfully following your diabetes health plan.

It may help to remember that people who question your results are doing so because they care about you. Of course, overlooking their remarks is easier said than done, especially when you feel like you are being interrogated. To handle the situation, you may want to:

■ Tell the person how it feels to be accused and that you honestly don't know why you aren't losing weight or your test results are high.
■ Honestly review your eating habits with yourself. Maybe you really are eating more than your meal plan allows but are not aware of it. Your physician and dietitian can help piece the mystery together.

If you find you are following your meal plan and you're not losing weight or aren't able to achieve good control with your present diabetes management plan, discuss it with your doctor. Together, you may be able to make some changes in your management plan.

checkups

(chek-UPS)

When you have diabetes, it pays to check—with your doctor, your eye doctor, and your podiatrist (a foot specialist, see Foot Care). You are the one responsible for day-to-day management of your diabetes, but it is your physician—through regular checkups—who can help make sure that your diabetes control efforts are on the right track.

How often should you have checkups? If you take insulin, a checkup every three months is recommended. If you are not taking insulin, a checkup every six months is recommended.

You should have an annual ophthalmic examination (a detailed eye examination) because retinopathy (see Retinopathy) can start to develop without noticeable symptoms. Early detection of eye problems can help prevent serious problems later. People with retinopathy may need more frequent visits.

Foot problems that seem minor can quickly become serious in people with diabetes. Every break in the skin of the foot of a person with diabetes should be taken seriously. Expect a thorough foot examination once or twice a year by your doctor or podiatrist.

What should you expect during your visits?

■ Eyes. Your doctor may check your eyes for any warning signs of retinopathy or refer you for regular visits to an ophthalmologist.

■ Feet. Each visit, your doctor should check the pulse in your feet and look for other signs of poor circulation, neuropathy, and infection.

■ Blood pressure. This should be checked on every visit. High blood pressure can increase a person's risk of developing heart, brain, eye, and kidney damage. High blood pressure can also make diabetes control very difficult.

■ Review of self-testing. Your doctor will want to know the results of both your blood and urine tests in order to make any needed changes in your routine. Your doctor may also order a glycohemoglobin test (see Blood Tests) to check your overall control since the last visit.

■ Weight. Dramatic changes could be either a result or cause of poor diabetes control. For children and adolescents, height should also be checked.

■ Complaints. Tell your doctor about any recurrent bouts of low blood sugar, symptoms of poor control (excessive thirst or urination), or any new symptoms (headache or blurred vision).

cholesterol

(ko-LESS-tur-awl)

Cholesterol, a white powder in pure form, is essential to good health. However, eating too much cholesterol can cause cholesterol in the blood to increase. Our bodies use cholesterol as a normal building block of the cell walls and also to make certain vitamins and hormones. It also helps form compounds called bile salts that aid digestion.

Cholesterol is found in all foods from animals, but is absent in food from plants. Though we get much of our cholesterol from the foods we eat, our livers have the ability to make enough cholesterol for our body's needs.

We get into trouble when we eat foods high in cholesterol, such as egg yolks, red meats, and organ meats (such as liver), because these may increase blood cholesterol levels. Foods rich in saturated fats are big culprits when it comes to containing cholesterol. Also, eating saturated fats causes blood cholesterol to increase. Saturated fats are found in such things as lard, dairy products, and certain vegetable oils like palm and coconut oil. Saturated fats are found mostly in foods from animals while unsaturated fats are found in foods from plants (see Fats).

Why is high blood cholesterol bad for you? It causes the most harm when it collects on the inner walls of a blood vessel. Eventually, this collection of cholesterol, along with other substances, can get so thick that it restricts or even cuts off blood flow—and causes a heart attack or stroke.

We don't want this to happen to you, so take our advice: In order to keep your blood cholesterol low, keep your cholesterol intake to less than 300 milligrams (mg) per day. (Most Americans consume between 400 to 500 mg a day.) You can do this by limiting your intake of fats so that no more than 30 percent of your total calories come from fat. In particular, you'll want to limit saturated fats.

Most people with diabetes can control their blood cholesterol by following the kind of diet that's been recom-

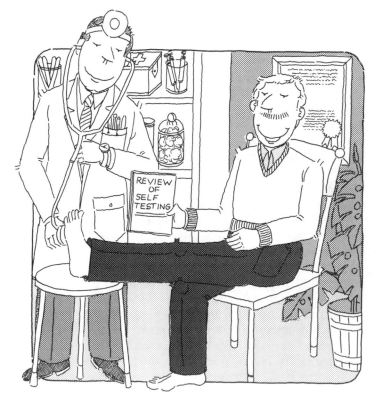

REVIEW OF SELF TESTING

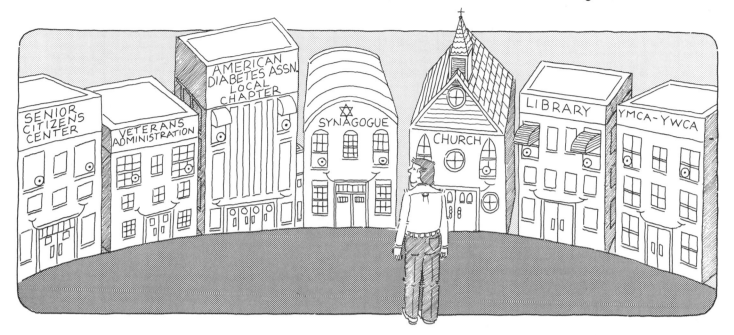

mended by the American Diabetes Association for controlling diabetes. Now that's easy, since you are already in the habit of good diabetes control. Right?

cold feet
(KOLD FEET)

Your cold feet may well be a sign of poor circulation or difficulties with nerve function in the feet. Warm them *only* by wearing socks. *Never* use a hot water bottle, bathe in hot water, or apply a heating pad to your feet. If you have diabetic neuropathy (nerve impairment) you can burn your feet without realizing it.

Other symptoms of poor circulation in your legs or feet include cramps in your calves when you walk and the loss of hair from the top of the feet. Discuss any symptoms of poor circulation with your physician and podiatrist so that treatment can be started promptly, before the circulation problem becomes too severe.

coma
(KO-mah)

Confused by the term "coma?" You are not alone. People generally think of a coma as an unconscious state. But then they hear doctors referring to a patient who is still conscious as having "diabetic coma." And then at other times, doctors may describe an insulin reaction as a form of "coma." And there are other forms of coma marked by high blood-glucose levels. Can any sense be made of all this?

The problem is that the term "coma" can either mean something very general or very specific. The general set of symptoms described by "coma" may include dizziness, disorientation, confusion, and possibly, unconsciousness. One or more of these symptoms may arise in a number of con-

ditions associated with diabetes. (See Hyperosmolar Coma, Insulin Reactions, and Ketoacidosis.)

Most often, however, the term "diabetic coma" refers specifically to *ketoacidosis*, a potentially life-threatening condition brought about by a lack of insulin. Ketoacidosis usually comes on gradually and is marked by prolonged high blood sugar and ketones in the urine. (To distinguish between ketoacidosis and insulin reactions, see the chart under the heading Warning Signs.)

community services
(ko-MYOO-ni-tee SUR-vis-es)

Besides your family and your health-care team, there are a wide range of community services that may be able to help you meet your particular needs.

For example, if you are having difficulty coping with diabetes or other problems, you may want to talk to a counselor. Your local church or synagogue may be able to meet your emotional needs. Or check the Yellow Pages of your phone book under "Social Service Organizations," for organizations that may be able to help you.

A big part of managing your diabetes is learning all you can about the disease. Your local American Diabetes Association affiliate or chapter is a great resource to help you continue your education about diabetes and find local support groups.

Also, don't forget your local library. The librarians there may be able to help you find information on any subject you are interested in, or at least be able to guide you to where you can find what you're looking for.

If you have served in the armed services, the Veterans Administration may be able to meet some of your needs, especially in health-related problems. (Check the U.S. government section of your phone book under "Veterans Administration.")

If you are ill and unable to leave your home, there are ser-

complications

vices that can help take care of your health as well as other needs such as shopping and housekeeping. (See Home Health Care.)

Whatever your problems or needs are, remember there are people in your community who can help. Don't feel you have to face problems alone—take advantage of the many resources available to you.

complications
(KOM-pli-KA-shuns)

Besides all the difficulties of properly taking care of your diabetes, there are other things you may have to deal with—complications. There are many things you can do in addition to controlling blood sugar to prevent complications from interfering with your normal activities.

The *acute* complications are those that can occur any time and can usually be corrected. These include *hypoglycemia* (low blood glucose), which is generally caused by too much insulin or oral antihypoglycemic pills (in relation to food and exercise), and *ketoacidosis* (coma), generally caused by a lack of insulin.

The long-term complications, which may take decades to develop, include small-blood-vessel disorders such as *retinopathy* (an eye disease that, in its advanced stages, can lead to blindness) and *nephropathy* (kidney disease). Unfortunately, long-term complications also include disorders of the nerves known as *neuropathies* (nerve damage) and disorders of the large blood vessels in the heart and elsewhere in the body. Blood-vessel disorders can impair blood circulation. Poor circulation in the feet combined with neuropathy sets the stage for the development of severe infections and gangrene.

Research appears to indicate that poor control may speed the development of complications; however, despite their best efforts, some people will develop complications anyway. Research also suggests that taking good control of your diabetes may help you to slow or even prevent these long-term complications. Genes (which determine characteristics a person inherits) are suspected of making some people more prone than others to complications.

No one can deny that the development of long-term diabetes complications is traumatic. However, treatments are usually available to treat or control the problems that develop. Regular checkups, to catch signs of changes early, are the best way to lessen the chances of developing complications.

If you do not have complications, you are wise to take all the steps you can to avoid developing them in the first place. Once complications develop they may be around to stay.

control
(kon-TROL)

Good diabetes control means keeping your blood-glucose levels as near to normal (nondiabetic) levels as possible.

You can do this by balancing diet, exercise, and insulin or oral medications.

Basically, this balance is doing for your body what a person's body without diabetes does automatically. You need to understand your body's needs and coordinate your schedule of meals, activities, and medication to avoid complications (your health-care team will help with this coordination). Studies have shown that elevated levels of blood glucose over a period of time can cause blood vessel damage. This damage can lead to complications in the eyes, kidneys, and nerves.

Blood-glucose and urine-ketone testing are important tools in diabetes control. Many people test their blood glucose two to four times a day and keep a record of their glucose levels. This record makes balancing food, exercise, and medication a lot easier.

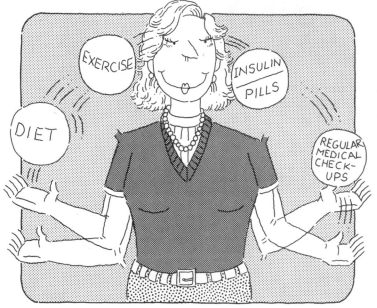

Ask your doctor how often you should test and how to use the test results to adjust food, exercise, and medications. Urine tests are much less accurate in determining glucose levels but play a necessary role in recognizing ketones. Ketones in your urine are a warning sign that ketoacidosis (diabetic coma) could occur. By testing your urine for ketones when you have a cold or the flu or when your blood glucose is more than 250 mg/dl, you may be able to take measures that will prevent ketoacidosis from happening or becoming more severe. (See Ketoacidosis.)

Controlling your diabetes also means regular checkups with your doctor. By reviewing your daily glucose records, your doctor can help you better manage your diabetes. And good diabetes management has its own reward: you will look and feel better.

C-peptide
(SEE-PEP-tide)

As far as researchers can tell, our bodies find the connecting peptide (or C-peptide) totally worthless. But diabetes researchers have discovered that the C-peptide is a valuable resource in determining how much insulin a pancreas produces.

In your pancreas, there are insulin-making cells called beta cells. These cells start out by making a large, coil-shaped molecule called proinsulin. This molecule is then chopped into two: one is insulin and the other is a small protein strand called the C-peptide.

Insulin plays an important role in regulating levels of glucose. C-peptide, however, doesn't seem to do much of anything for the body. Researchers and doctors, though, find C-peptide very useful—especially in helping to distinguish between type I (insulin-dependent) diabetes and type II (non-insulin-dependent) diabetes. For every insulin molecule made, there is also a molecule of C-peptide. Both are secreted into the bloodstream in equal amounts. This allows researchers to determine how much insulin is being made in the pancreas.

Why can't you just measure the amount of insulin in the blood? Only about half of all the insulin made is circulated in the blood. After insulin leaves the pancreas, it is scooped up by the liver. The C-peptide, however, gets through the liver untouched. Thus, the amount of C-peptide in the blood reflects the amount of insulin made by the pancreas.

The test to determine a person's C-peptide level can be performed in most hospitals and commercial laboratories. This test helps determine the level of insulin a person's body is producing. Some people treated with insulin (those with type II diabetes) actually have enough insulin of their own. Sometimes the C-peptide level may be tested to see if a person's body is producing insulin on its own. If the C-peptide level is normal, it is possible a person's diabetes could be managed with supplemental insulin, along with meal planning and weight loss. If the C-peptide level is low, it is likely the person has type I (insulin-dependent) diabetes, and will need regular insulin injections.

If you have non-insulin-dependent (type II) diabetes your doctor might be interested in measuring your C-peptide level. Unlike people with type I diabetes, who always have a shortage of insulin, type II people may make low, normal, or even high levels of insulin. Results from this test may help your doctor choose a proper treatment plan for managing your diabetes. The test is also useful to researchers studying new treatment plans and ways to prevent diabetes.

dating
(DAY-ting)

There's no reason why diabetes should hold you back from dating. Dating is just one more life experience to look forward to with excitement.

Some people wonder if they should tell their date they have diabetes. The fact is, it's usually easier to bring it out in the open—but make sure *you* choose the time; don't let it choose you. In other words, don't wait for an insulin reaction.

Telling your date you have diabetes is especially helpful if you plan to eat at a restaurant or at someone's house. This way, you can discuss the timing of your meal without seeming like a pathological stickler for punctuality. If you are going to

someone's house for dinner, you may want to find out what is on the menu beforehand, so you won't be caught off guard by "forbidden" foods.

If you want to bring a snack during a date without making a big deal out of it, bring enough to share. Be creative with your snack, and let your knowledge of good foods impress your date.

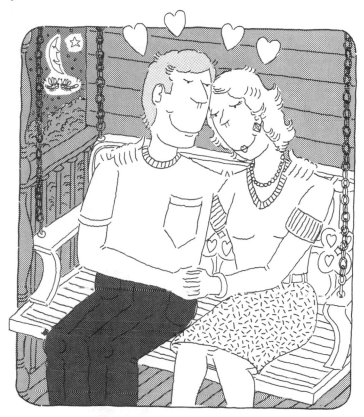

Have you ever worried that someone might not want to date you because you have diabetes? Don't jump to conclusions. Diabetes is often used as an excuse for many things, including being turned down for a date. Of course, if someone does have a hangup about your diabetes, it's *their* hangup—not yours. Remember that most people tend to accept diabetes the same way the person who has it does. If you feel comfortable with it, so will others.

Sometimes it's not your date, but one or both of your date's parents who have second thoughts about your diabetes. If they don't know about diabetes, try to explain it to them, but don't be hostile about it. Your good attitude toward diabetes—and the fact that you lead a normal life—will say more than any words ever could.

Of course, how much you tell your date about your diabetes (if in fact you do choose to talk about it) is up to you. But if the relationship seems to be getting serious it's time to sit down and share your understanding and feelings about diabetes. Don't be surprised if your partner goes through some of the same emotional stages—such as anger, denial, and adjustment—that you went through when you first learned you had diabetes. It will take some time for the two of you to learn how to work diabetes into your lives, instead of having it *define* them.

dawn phenomenon

(DAWN fe-NOM-ah-NON)

If you have diabetes, you may find that it's not just the sun that rises at dawn. Many people with diabetes experience what researchers call the dawn phenomenon—an unexpected increase in blood sugar between the hours of 4 a.m. and 8 a.m.

These early-morning surges aren't unique to people with diabetes. In a study, researchers found that people without diabetes also experience rises in their blood-glucose levels early in the morning. To compensate, their insulin levels also rise. Researchers have concluded that the dawn phenomenon is related to the body's behavior during sleep. It seems the body naturally releases more glucose in the early morning as it is waking up. This increase in glucose signals the need for more insulin. But in diabetes, either the pancreas can't meet the demand for insulin or the body can't use the insulin properly. So, on waking, your blood-glucose level is high.

While not all reasons behind the dawn phenomenon have been discovered, the search has been narrowed to the growth hormone. This hormone is secreted in spurts right after sleep begins. However, it takes about six hours for the growth hormone to raise blood sugar; this explains why blood sugar rises in the morning. A person's growth hormone secretion varies from night to night which is why the dawn phenomenon is so difficult to predict and control. Also, the dawn phenomenon is usually most severe for people during adolescence and early adulthood—when the growth hormone is at its peak.

If you are experiencing high blood glucose in the early morning, you and your doctor will want to look at your treatment plan to find the cause. Before diagnosing the dawn phenomenon, two explainable causes for high blood glucose will need to be eliminated. They are: not enough insulin to cover your body's need for the night, or problems with insulin reactions and rebound.

To rule out these two possible causes, your doctor may ask you to test your blood glucose some mornings at 3 a.m. If your blood glucose is on the high end of normal or high, you probably do not have enough insulin to cover your body's needs. Treatment for this problem then would be to increase your insulin dosage. If, on the other hand, your blood sugar is on the low end of normal or low at 3 a.m., you probably are taking too much insulin and are experiencing rebound. (See Rebound.)

Once these two common causes of high blood sugar have been treated or ruled out, dawn phenomenon will move into place as the prime suspect. Despite any attempts you or your doctor make, you still may be unable to avoid these high blood sugar surges. But research into the dawn phenomenon and viable treatments is on-going, and there is hope that sometime in the future, you'll be able to start every day in control.

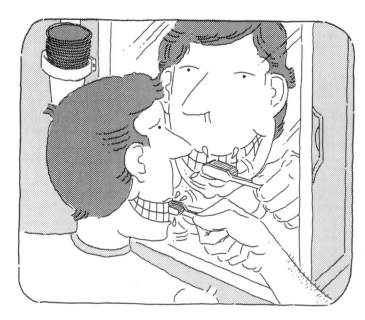

DCCT

(Diabetes Control and Complications Trial)

The Diabetes Control and Complications Trial (DCCT) is the largest and most comprehensive clinical experiment ever conducted in diabetes research. This study, backed by the National Institutes of Health, is being conducted in 27 research centers in the United States and Canada to study the benefits of tight control (keeping blood glucose as close to normal—nondiabetic—levels as possible).

For years, doctors have speculated that tight control of diabetes can prevent or postpone many of the complications of diabetes and the DCCT is being conducted to see if this is so.

Hundreds of volunteers throughout North America are being studied. One group will follow an intensive treatment regimen: They will use three or more insulin injections a day or will use an insulin pump. The second group will follow the traditional treatment of one or two insulin injections a day. Both groups will be closely monitored.

The study is not expected to be completed until 1993 or 1994.

dental care

(DEN-tall KARE)

Don't you just hate to go to the dentist? Well, if you don't keep your diabetes under control you may dislike that visit even more—poor control increases your chances of losing your teeth to *periodontal disease.*

Cavities aren't the only threat to our teeth. Periodontal disease, gum infections that occur around the teeth, plays a major role in tooth loss. The first stage of periodontal disease is *gingivitis.* This is where the gums become inflamed because plaque (a film that forms on your teeth from food, saliva, and bacteria) has been allowed to build up on the teeth near the gums. Some signs of gingivitis include mild inflammation—slight redness and swelling of gum tissue around one or more teeth. Daily flossing and brushing can help prevent plaque from collecting on your teeth.

Plaque that is not removed through daily brushing and flossing, hardens and turns into calculus, or tartar. This tartar extends from the gum line down around the root of the tooth irritating the gums. Disease sets in as bacteria builds up around the gums. If left untreated, the gums eventually shrink away from the tooth and form a pocket. As the infection spreads, pus may form, like it forms when any irritation, such as a splinter, infects and destroys tissue. Eventually, the ligaments holding the roots of the tooth to the bone are destroyed and the tooth loosens and may be lost.

If you notice that your gums bleed easily, especially when you are brushing your teeth, you may have some early signs of gum disease. In more advanced stages of gum disease, you may notice one or more of your teeth are lose or have shifted. Also, you may notice pus coming out of your gums when you press them. If you notice any of these signs, you should visit your dentist.

About 85 percent of Americans over the age of 40 suffer from some form of periodontal disease. Recent studies have shown that people with diabetes are at higher risk for developing *periodontitis*, the more severe form of gum disease. Periodontal disease is often more frequent and more severe in people with diabetes and tends to appear at an earlier age. You can reduce the risk of gingivitis or periodontitis by keeping your diabetes in control.

You look a lot better with your own pearly whites and should do what you can to keep them. Here are a few suggestions:

■ Keep your diabetes under control. Well-controlled blood-glucose levels are the most important step you can take to prevent tooth and gum problems.
■ See your dentist for a checkup at least once every six months. Be sure to tell your dentist you have diabetes. Ask your dentist to show you how to better take care of your teeth.
■ Brush at least twice a day. Use a soft-bristle brush between the gums and the teeth in a vibrating motion.
■ Be sure to floss daily. Ask your dentist to show you how.
■ If you need treatment for periodontal disease, you should first be evaluated by your physician. If diabetes is poorly controlled, most treatment for advanced periodontal disease should be delayed until better control is established.

depression

(de-PRESH-un)

There is no denying it—diabetes can be depressing. If you have been recently diagnosed, taking control of diabetes may seem too much to handle all of a sudden and you may get the blues. You may feel singled out or different from other people and that may make you sad. Or guilt from not staying true to your treatment plan may drop your spirits.

Whatever the reason, we all have times when nothing seems to be going right and we get depressed. In fact, a little sadness can often help us in the long run by making us think

about a situation and learn how to better handle it next time. While the day-to-day handling of diabetes can bring you down at times, the blues shouldn't dominate your life. Here are some ways to get out of the dumps:

■ Keep active. Pursue interests, hobbies, leisure activities, sports, exercise, and arts and crafts.
■ Stay in touch with family and friends. Invite them to join you in activities you enjoy.
■ Don't dwell on the negative or minimize the positive. No one is perfect; a bad experience doesn't mean you're a failure. Remember to acknowledge your accomplishments.
■ Take responsibility for both your failures and successes. You can feel better by apologizing when you think you're wrong. But don't assume responsibility or guilt for events beyond your control.
■ Don't set unrealistic expectations for yourself. Just do your best and take satisfaction in trying your hardest.
■ Don't give up. Also, don't hesitate to seek help when you think you need it from a professional counselor who can help you in coping with the stresses of daily living.

If your depression lingers on for a long period of time, you may be suffering from serious clinical depression. If this is the case, you need to seek professional help. Some of these symptoms are:

■ Sad, hopeless mood, and loss of interest or pleasure in usual activities.
■ Before psychiatrists and other health professionals diagnose serious depression they look for at least four of the following to occur almost daily for at least two weeks:
■ Poor appetite and weight loss or increased appetite and noticeable weight gain.
■ Sleep disturbances—either getting too little or too much sleep.
■ Loss of interest in sex.
■ Loss of energy, constant fatigue.
■ Feelings of worthlessness, self-blame, and guilt.
■ Problems in concentrating, remembering, and decision-making.
■ Repeated thoughts of death and suicide.

diabetes

(DI-a-BEET-eez)

In a nutshell, diabetes is a disease in which the body does not produce or respond to insulin (a hormone produced by the pancreas). Without insulin, your body cannot properly convert the food you eat into energy. Energy is necessary to performing the daily tasks of life. Diabetes (more properly, *diabetes mellitus*) is actually a general term for a number of separate but related disorders. These disorders fall into two main categories: type I and type II.

People with type I (insulin-dependent) diabetes produce little or no insulin—the hormone that "unlocks" the cells of the body, allowing glucose to enter and fuel them. Without insulin, glucose simply builds up in the blood. (Eventually, it "spills over" into the urine.) While glucose is building up in the blood, the body's cells literally starve to death. So

dieting

people with type I diabetes must take daily insulin injections to stay alive. They also need to balance the injections with a carefully prescribed regimen of food and exercise to keep blood sugar within an acceptable range.

Type I diabetes generally, but not always, occurs in childhood or adolescence, which is why it was once called "juvenile diabetes." An estimated one million individuals—5 to 15 percent of all people with diabetes—have this form of the disease.

Symptoms of type I diabetes, which usually develop suddenly, include:

- extreme thirst
- frequent urination
- inability to gain weight regardless of food intake
- nausea
- weakness and fatigue
- irritability
- extreme hunger, especially for sweets

Type II (non-insulin-dependent) diabetes occurs most often in people past age 40. This is why it was formally called adult-onset or maturity-onset diabetes. Still, anyone at any age could have type II diabetes. Many people don't realize they have type II diabetes because it develops gradually and the symptoms are not always recognized easily. Many times the symptoms are confused with the aging process and are ignored. The fact that few people with type II diabetes need to take insulin has led to the notion that this is a "mild" form of the disease. But type II diabetes should be taken seriously. Left unchecked, type II can lead to the same long-term complications—including retinopathy, kidney disease, and atherosclerosis—that can occur among people with type I diabetes.

About 90 percent of all people who have type II diabetes are overweight. Other people are not overweight but their bodies react as if they were. These people may look thin but in reality have more body fat than muscle. Another group of people are actually thin but for some unknown reason their pancreases don't produce enough insulin to meet their bodies' needs. Still, another group may have type II because of a combination of these problems.

Researchers do not quite understand the correlation between obesity and type II diabetes. For most people with type II, the problem is not so much being able to produce enough insulin but rather being able to use insulin efficiently. And it seems, for reasons unknown, that excess fat makes it more difficult for a person's body to use insulin efficiently.

To understand this problem, we need to look at the body's cells. The cells of the body have insulin receptors. These are "keyholes" on the surface of the cells into which insulin—the "key"—fits. Insulin "unlocks" the cells, allowing glucose to enter. Apparently, people with type II diabetes either don't have enough insulin receptors, or the receptors aren't working properly. The result, the same as in type I diabetes, is that glucose has a hard time getting into the cells.

Often, type II diabetes can be controlled through dieting and exercise (which lowers blood sugar) alone. But sometimes, these are not enough. Many people with type II diabetes also need to take medication (either oral diabetes

medicine or insulin).

Any of the symptoms listed above for type I diabetes may also be a sign of type II. Additional symptoms include:

- slow healing of cuts and other injuries
- frequent skin, gum, or urinary infections
- blurred vision
- pain in legs, hands, or feet
- itching
- drowsiness

As with the symptoms of type I diabetes, any one of these problems might be the initial tip-off that a person has diabetes. If you recognize any of these signs in yourself, see your physician.

Two other kinds of diabetes that are less common are gestational diabetes and impaired glucose tolerance. For a discussion on these, look under the headings for each.

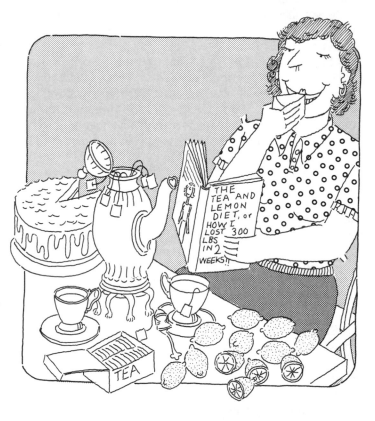

dieting
(DI-et-ing)

Grapefruit diet. Watermelon diet. Lemon and tea diet . . .you've heard all about the fantastic weight loss people have achieved following weird diets such as these. What you don't hear is that two weeks or two months later all those "lost" pounds somehow are "found" again.

Dieting—the act of restricting the number of calories you eat—has earned a bad, and potentially dangerous, name because people want to lose weight quickly.

There are many fad diets on the market that claim to offer quick and easy weight loss. Most, if not all of these, should be avoided. Check with your doctor. Diets that are particularly dangerous to your health are those that are low in calories or rely on a limited variety of foods—for example, those that limit your diet to only fruits and proteins.

When you limit yourself to only 500 to 1,000 calories a day or do not include a good variety of foods in your diet, your body does not get all the nutrients it needs. That is why this kind of diet should only be done under a doctor's supervision, and the doctor would likely prescribe vitamin and mineral supplements.

Even under a doctor's supervision, the kind of diet just mentioned is not recommended for most people. The best way to lose and control your weight is to balance the amount of food you eat with your level of activity—in other words, meal planning and exercise.

Both meal planning and exercise are not only good for weight control; they are essential to good diabetes control. (See Exercise and Meal Planning.) Work with your doctor or dietitian to develop a meal plan that works for you. If the first one doesn't work, ask for a consultation to find out why, and how to make the right adjustments. Also, talk with your doctor about exercises that you'll be able to participate in—both because you want to *and* because they're safe for you.

Like anything worthwhile, effective meal planning and exercise will be a challenge. But once you get used to the routine and start feeling and seeing the results of a healthy lifestyle, you'll find effective weight control well worth the effort.

digestion

(di-JES-ton)

You open your mouth. You place the fork on your tongue and close your jaw so your teeth grab the food. You chew. You swallow. . .but then, what *really* happens?

Formally, it's called digestion. This process starts as soon as your nose smells food and can end 24, 48, or even 72 hours later—after your body has thoroughly processed the food stuffs and then disposes of the unused leftovers.

Digestion occurs after food has been chewed, mixed with the saliva in your mouth, and swallowed. From the mouth, the food travels down the esophagus (the tube that leads from the mouth down to the stomach). In the stomach, acids are secreted that break down the food. After the food has been broken down sufficiently, it is passed to the small intestine. There, nutrients and water are taken out to serve the body's nutritional needs. The remaining food—particularly fiber—is then passed to the large intestine where more water is removed. From the large intestine, the "leftovers" enter the rectum where they are stored until they can be excreted. (Sometimes, damage to the autonomic nerves will weaken the effectiveness of your digestive tract. See Neuropathy.)

Pretty exhausting process your body goes through to digest your food, isn't it? Well, next time you decide to go on an eating binge, think about all the work your body would have to go through. Then, turn to your meal plan and give your digestive system a break.

driving

(DRIV-ing)

No state in America prevents people from driving solely because they have diabetes. However, some states may require a medical statement showing your diabetes is in good control and that you don't suffer from any complications that would interfere with your driving.

Getting a license, however, is just the first requirement for being a safe driver. For your own security—and that of others—take the following precautions:

■ Do not drive if you feel an insulin reaction coming on. If you are unsure, test your blood. When you cannot test, cover yourself by having some simple carbohydrate before you drive. Better yet, ask someone else to take the wheel.

■ Keep sugary food or drink (such as juice in a can) handy at all times. If you feel a reaction coming on while driving, pull over as soon as safely possible and drink your juice or eat your food.

■ If you will be driving at the same time your insulin will be peaking, eat a snack before you set off. This is also good advice for people who have difficulty recognizing that a reaction is coming on. (If you have a problem recognizing a reaction, be sure to talk to your doctor. He or she may be able to help you recognize a reaction and help you to take better precautions.)

■ If you feel ill or tired from high blood sugar or other fac-

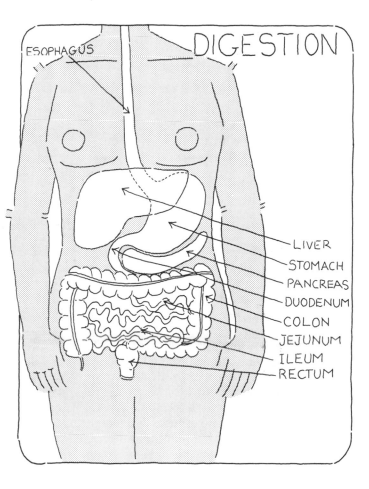

drugs

tors, do not drive.

■ If neuropathy has made your feet numb, do not drive. You may not have good control over the gas and brake pedals.

■ Do not drink and drive.

■ Wear and carry identification at all times which states that you have diabetes.

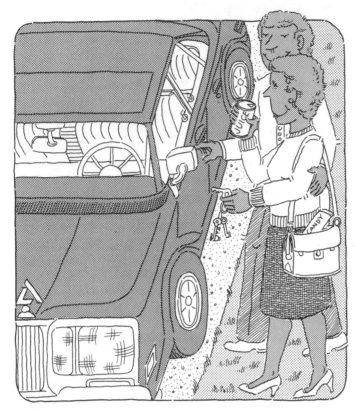

drugs
(DRUGS)

Knowing how to use medicines safely is important—and not just for people with diabetes. Anyone who cares about his or her health has a responsibility to know what a medication is doing inside the body. By not knowing the rules of safe drug use, a person can be an easy mark for a variety of drug-related problems:

■ Drug allergies. Many people are allergic to certain drugs (penicillin is a well-known example). The allergic reaction can be as mild as a rash or as serious as *something called an anaphylactic shock*, a condition where the body violently reacts to a substance it recognizes as foreign. This reaction can result in life-threatening effects, such as loss of blood pressure and heart rate. Usually another, nonallergic, drug can be substituted.

■ Side effects. A single drug seldom has just a single effect on the body. Antihistamines, for example, in addition to drying your sinuses, may make you drowsy or can increase the effects of alcohol in your system. The strength of a drug's side effects varies from person to person.

■ Drug interactions. Two or more different drugs, working in the body at the same time, can interfere with each other's actions. They might boost each other's strength, cancel each

other out, or combine to produce a new—and probably undesirable—effect. Some drugs can also interact with alcohol or even certain foods. One example is monoamine oxidase (MAO) inhibitors. MAO inhibitors are prescribed for depression, but can cause violent, even fatal, reactions when taken together with bleu cheese. (These reactions happen because of the effects the MAO inhibitors have on normal nerve stimulation in blood vessels.)

■ Unheeded instructions. When it comes to drugs, too much of a good thing can spell trouble (as anyone who takes insulin well knows). Not enough of a good thing can be equally risky. If the instructions on a bottle of antibiotics say to keep taking the drug even after you start feeling better, keep taking it. If you don't, your ailment may well return in full fury (but do talk to your doctor about adjusting your dosage).

People with diabetes have additional concerns. You need to know whether a drug will affect your blood-glucose level, either by raising it or lowering it. If you use oral diabetes medicine, you also need to know whether a new drug will interact with your medicine. Few drugs are absolutely forbidden for people with diabetes, but if they have an effect on blood-glucose levels, that effect must be taken into account. You may need to talk with your doctor about readjusting your treatment plan.

A word of warning about over-the-counter drugs (the kind you don't need a prescription to purchase): Watch out for those that contain sugar (such as cough drops and syrups). Ask your pharmacist whether a drug comes in a sugarless form.

Many over-the-counter cold pills and diet pills contain ingredients (such as ephedrine and phenylpropanolamine) that can raise blood sugar and wreak havoc on diabetes control. These drugs should never be used without checking with your doctor.

On the other hand, large amounts of aspirin taken for chronic pain can lower your blood-glucose levels. Most people with diabetes can take aspirin, but its effects on blood glucose should be monitored. Ask your doctor if you can safely take aspirin.

The accompanying chart shows many of the major prescription drugs that may have an effect on blood glucose. Those drugs listed in **bold type** can have particularly severe effects. But remember that drugs act differently in different people. The same drug may raise blood glucose sharply in one person with diabetes, while affecting another only slightly or not at all. Your best bet? Check with your doctor before taking any drug.

eating out
(EAT-ing OUT)

Part of the fun of eating out is sampling cuisine you wouldn't cook at home. Don't deny yourself these adventures in dining. If you've learned your meal plan and exchanges, you should have little difficulty choosing interesting dishes

drugs that can affect blood-sugar levels

GENERIC NAME	COMMON BRAND NAMES	EFFECT ON BLOOD-SUGAR LEVELS	INTERACTS WITH ORAL MEDICATION	COMMON USES
Anabolic Steriods	Dianabol	Lowers	No	Increasing muscle mass.
Chloramphenicol	Chloromycetin	Lowers*	Yes	Potent antibiotic.
Corticosteriods	Prednisone, Decadron, Kenalog, Cortisone	Raises	Yes	Treating inflammation, redness, and swelling in a variety of disorders.
Coumarin Anticoagulants	Dicumarol	Lowers*	Yes	Preventing blood clots.
Diazoxide	Hyperstat, Proglycem	Raises	Yes	Treating low blood sugar caused by pancreatic tumors; also sometimes used for treating hypertension.
Diuretics	Diuril, HydroDIURIL, Esidrix, Diamox	Raises	Yes	Relieves fluid buildup by increasing volume of urine.
Epinephrine, Adrenaline	Adrenalin	Raises	Yes	Reviving heartbeat; treating severe allergic reactions.
Estrogens, Birth Control Pills	(sold under several brand names	Raises	No	Preventing pregnancy and also to lessen the effects of menopause.
Fenfluramine	Pondimin	Lowers	No	An appetite suppressant.
Lithium Carbonate	Eskalith, Lithane	Raises	No	Treating manic-depressive illness.
Methyldopa	Aldomet	Lowers*	Yes	Treating high blood pressure.
Monoamine Oxidase Inhibitors, MAO Inhibitors	Parnate, Nardil, Eutonyl	Lowers	Yes	Used in treating severe depression
Nicontinic Acid, Niacin	Nicolar, Nicobid	Raises	No	Nutrition suplement; also sometimes used to treat high cholesterol levels.
Phenobarbital	Solfoton	Raises*	Yes	Sedative; also sometimes used in treating epilepsy.
Phenylbutazone	Butazolidin	Lowers*	Yes	Treating arthritis.
Phenytoin	Dilantin	Raises	Yes	Treating epilepsy and other nervous-system disorders.
Propanolol	Inderal	Lowers† or Raises	No	Treating angina, unsteady heartbeats, overactive thyroids, and other ailments.
Rifampin	Rifadin	Raises*	Yes	Treating tuberculosis.
Sulfa Drugs	Gantrisin, Septra, Bactrim	Lowers*	Yes	Antiobiotics.
Thyroid Preparations, Desiccated Thyroid		Raises	No	Used to compensate for thyroid deficiency.

These drugs raise or lower blood sugar only *when used in combination with oral diabetes medicine.*

†*Propanolol generally lowers blood sugar but in some people, primarily those with Type II diabetes, it can* raise *it.*

entertaining

wherever you go. Here are some tips for taking the worry out of eating out:

■ Become familiar with serving sizes by practicing at home. As you practice with the right amount of food that fits your meal plan, you will learn to recognize what correct portions look like in the restaurant.

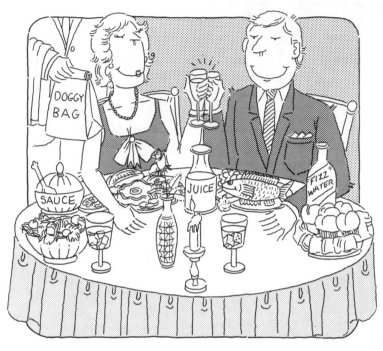

■ Don't plow into a meal that has generous restaurant-sized portions. If you are served an eight-ounce steak, start the meal by cutting it in half and asking for a doggie bag for half of it. If the potato is a hefty Idaho that takes up a quarter of your plate, do the same with it. You'll have a free meal for the next day.

■ Have salad dressing, margarine, sour cream, or sauces served "on the side."

■ Ask specific questions about how food is prepared. And opt for broiled foods whenever possible. If something you want isn't on the menu, ask for it.

■ Avoid fried or fatty foods, sauces, and sweet desserts. Avoid casseroles and stews—better to eat these at home so you know what's in them.

■ Good selections include meats in which the fat has been trimmed and the gravy has been omitted, and salads with no dressing.

■ Eat on schedule. If you think there might be a delay, eat part of your usual meal before going to the restaurant.

entertaining

(EN-ter-TANE-ing)

Do you feel you have to cook one way for yourself and a different way for company? Nonsense! The cooking and eating habits you've developed to help manage your diabetes are healthy habits for everybody—so don't think you've lost your touch as a host/hostess.

Of course, if your guests are traditional meat/fat lovers, they may choose to eat what you serve in different proportions than you do. So you may choose to be prepared to serve slightly larger portions than you would eat yourself. If you wind up with leftovers, freeze them and have them later.

When you bring the main course to the table, let service be family-style, with everyone serving their own portions. This is a good way to serve food because you can take less than your guests of given items, and they'll be less likely to notice since they'll be serving themselves. If you don't cook with salt, be sure to have some available on the table for your guests who use it.

What about hors d'oeuvres? Try cutting up carrots, celery, broccoli, cauliflower, and green peppers into bite-sized strips. Add cherry tomatoes. Instead of a dip high in fat, try low fat yogurt or blender-whipped cottage cheese for a base. Then add curry powder to one bowl, dill and pepper to another, and horseradish and minced onion to a third. Your guests will gobble them up.

Everyone loves dessert, but don't feel like you have to serve a Black Forest cake or mud pie to be considered a perfect hostess. Turn to fruits for wonderfully sweet desserts without adding sugar. For example, simmer sliced apples in orange juice with a few cinnamon sticks until the apples are soft. You won't believe the sweet taste, and your guests will never guess there is no added sugar.

You can find more tips on entertaining and lots of great recipes in the American Diabetes Association's *Family Cookbook* (Volumes I, II, III, and IV) and *Holiday Cookbook*. Check with your affiliate for more information (see the white pages of your phone book).

exchanges

(eks-CHANJ-es)

The exchange system for meal planning isn't difficult to understand— once you understand what the "exchanges" are and how they work. An "exchange" simply means a trade or substitute. The Exchange List system was devised by the American Diabetes Association and The American Dietetic Association to simplify meal planning. Here's how it works:

All foods are placed in one of six basic groups: Starch/Bread, Meat and Meat Substitutes, Vegetables, Fruit, Milk, and Fat. Any food in a given group can be exchanged for any other food in that group, in the amount shown. For example, a small apple can be exchanged for a small orange. A half cup of asparagus is equal to, and can be exchanged for, a half cup of zucchini. An ounce of lean beef can be exchanged for an ounce of fish. And so on.

People often wonder why peas are listed under Starch/Bread exchanges (instead of Vegetable) and cheeses are listed under Meat exchanges (instead of Milk). The reason is that foods are placed into exchange groups because they are alike—each selection contains about the same amount of carbohydrate, protein, calories, and fat. For example, the protein, carbohydrate, and fat content of a starchy vegetable like peas is closer to that of breads and cereals than to vegetables, like green beans. Similarly, the nutrient content of cottage cheese is closer to that of tuna than a glass of milk. The accompanying chart shows how much of which kinds of nutrients go into each exchange group.

Once you have learned the foods in the six lists and can gauge the correct portion, you can vary your diet easily at home, in the homes of friends, in a restaurant, at the ballpark, or even the company picnic.

You can get a copy of the *Exchange Lists for Meal Planning* by contacting your local American Diabetes Association chapter or affiliate. Check the white pages of your telephone book for an affiliate near you.

exercise

(EK-ser-SIZE)

In the old days, when people worked in the field instead of behind a desk, getting enough exercise was not a major health concern. But in this computer age, where sedentary lives are contributing to diseases such as atherosclerosis, obesity, hypertension, and diabetes, exercise is a hot topic in terms of leading a healthy and productive life. In fact, along with diet and medication, exercise is one of the three major factors that contribute to proper diabetes control.

Exercise has several benefits. It improves circulation and muscle tone and can contribute to weight loss. Also, it can help you relieve tension, make you feel good, and look fit. While any exercise is beneficial, aerobic exercise is best. Aerobic exercise is continuous and rhythmical, such as bicycling, walking, swimming, running, skating, cross-country skiing, and rowing. It improves the flow of blood through the small blood vessels, increases the pumping power of the heart, and when done on a regular basis, slows the pulse rate. For people with diabetes who are prone to vascular (blood vessel) disease, the benefits of this type of exercise are one form of protection against heart trouble and blood vessel disease.

That is not the only benefit people with diabetes get from exercise: Unless diabetes is in poor control (very high blood sugar or the presence of ketones), exercise usually lowers blood-glucose levels. Exercise also seems to help the action of insulin. As blood glucose is lowered, the body uses food more efficiently and little or no sugar is lost in the urine.

What this means is that if you have type I diabetes, you need to plan your exercise routine in conjunction with your diet and the action times of your insulin. You should try to exercise after a meal when glucose is rising. If an unplanned exercise or physical activity comes up and your blood sugar is normal or low to begin with, you should eat a snack before you get going—half a sandwich should do it. This will help prevent having too much insulin and too little glucose circulating in the blood, which would result in an insulin reaction.

As a general rule, if you are going to participate in short-term or moderate exercise (such as golf, biking, or walking) you'll want to eat a high-carbohydrate snack. Some high-carbohydrate snacks are: bread, raisins or other fruit, and

exchange groups

List Name	Carbohydrates (grams)	Protein (grams)	Fat (grams)	Calories
Starch/Bread	15	3	trace	80
Meat				
Lean	—	7	3	55
Medium-fat	—	7	5	75
High-fat	—	7	8	100
Vegetable	5	2	—	25
Fruit	15	—	—	60
Milk				
Skim	12	8	trace	90
Low-fat	12	8	5	120
Whole	12	8	8	150
Fat	—	—	5	45

fruit juices. (One Fruit exchange plus one Starch/Bread exchange should be enough for moderate exercise. However, check with your doctor to see what he/she recommends.) If you're planning on doing more strenuous exercises for more than an hour, you may also want to eat a small amount of protein. (One ounce or one Meat exchange should be plenty.)

If you feel a reaction coming on while you are exercising, *stop*, and take some form of carbohydrate that is quickly absorbed by the body. (See Insulin Reaction.) Something like orange juice, sugar, or a non-diet soft drink should do the trick. If you participate in an activity such as running, you can take along a quick acting carbohydrate such as hard candy, glucose gel, or a sugar packet for when your blood glucose gets low.

If you're into team sports such as basketball, football, baseball, or soccer, you should let someone (a coach, or a team member) know you have diabetes and teach them how to help you, just in case you need their help.

You like individual sports such as running, bicycling, skiing, or hiking? Great! Just remember to avoid exercising alone. If you can, find a friend or family member to go along. Besides being a safety precaution, it will make the workout more enjoyable. If you can't find anyone and still want to exercise, let someone know where you are going and when you expect to get back. You'll need to test your blood sugar more often to be safe. Also, be sure to carry some food with you to treat an insulin reaction. And, remember to carry some identification which says that you have diabetes.

If you participate in exercise that is unusually heavy or prolonged, you may also find that you have hypoglycemic reactions several hours later, even the next day (see Hypoglycemia). This can usually be prevented by taking extra food, particularly carbohydrate, to help the body rebuild its

exercise

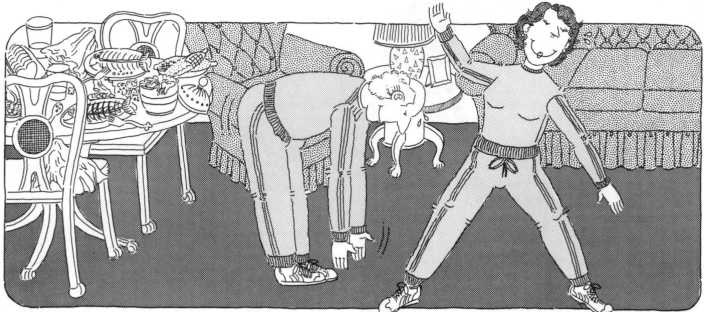

energy stores. In some situations when it is possible to anticipate prolonged or strenuous exercise, you may be able to cut back on your insulin dose to help prevent hypoglycemia. If this is a problem for you, discuss it with your doctor.

You're all excited to get started—right? Well, don't get so excited that you overdo it. Exercise is only beneficial when you do it properly. The first step is to check with your doctor before starting any exercise routine. Work with your doc-

tor to achieve the best control you can while exercising. So both you and your doctor can make adjustments in your treatment plan, keep track of your injections, the amount of insulin you inject, when and what you eat, and the times when you exercise. Also, test your blood sugar often and record the results. All this information will help you and your doctor achieve a balance between food, exercise and insulin.

Next, start out slowly and work up gradually. Make sure

burn those calories

ACTIVITY	CALORIES BURNED EACH MINUTE	CALORIES BURNED IN AN HOUR
Light housework, such as polishing furniture or washing small clothes.	2-2½	120-150
Golf, using power cart. Level walking at 2 miles per hour.	2½-4	150-240
Cleaning windows, mopping floors, or vacuuming. Walking at 3 miles per hour. Golf, pulling cart. Cycling at 6 miles per hour. Bowling.	4-5	240-300
Scrubbing floors. Cycling 8 miles per hour. Walking 3½ miles per hour. Table tennis, badminton, and volleyball. Doubles tennis. Golf, carrying clubs. Many calisthenics and ballet exercises.	5-6	300-360
Walking 4 miles per hour. Ice or roller skating. Cycling 10 miles per hour.	6-7	360-420
Walking 5 miles per hour. Cycling 11 miles per hour. Water skiing. Singles tennis.	7-8	420-480
Jogging 5 miles per hour. Cycling 12 miles per hour. Downhill skiing. Paddleball.	8-10	480-600
Running 5½ miles per hour. Cycling 13 miles per hour. Squash or handball (practice or warmup session).	10-11	600-660
Running 6 miles per hour or more. competitive handball or squash.	11 or more	660 or more

you choose the correct gear to fit the sport. When choosing a shoe, get one designed for the activity you want to participate in. Finally, keep your diabetes in control by carefully following your diet plan and insulin or pill dosage.

family involvement
(FAM-i-lee in-VOLV-ment)

Being diagnosed with diabetes is a traumatic experience for anyone. At first, it can be very difficult for the person to cope with the disease and the changes in lifestyle necessary to keep his or her diabetes in control. At the same time, family members may also have difficulty adjusting to the disease.

For one, changes in the preparation and timing of meals may pose special problems for all family members. For the person with diabetes, especially type I, the timing of a meal is all-important to good diabetes control. The family used to eating on a regular schedule won't find this threatening. However, the family whose mealtimes differ from day to day may have difficulty getting used to a routine. Similarly, the family who regularly eats well-balanced meals will be less affected by the dietary changes of diabetes than the family whose usual dinner consists of fast food and soft drinks.

Parents who have a child with diabetes may also face another challenge when it comes to providing snacks. The child with diabetes may feel left out when the other children in the family are allowed to eat "forbidden" foods. You, as a parent, may decide to resolve this problem by preparing healthy snacks for the whole family.

Another challenge for families is learning to balance "time" with a child who has diabetes and with those that don't. Some children may resent the "extra" attention being given the child with diabetes. This is normal. Parents may need to take time to give special attention to each child. Also, the nondiabetic children may fear their brother or sister with diabetes will die. They may also worry that they themselves will get diabetes. For this reason, parents may need to spend some time fully explaining diabetes to their nondiabetic children.

There are other challenges too. Family members may fear the complications of diabetes and their ability to handle them. Spouses may have feelings of resentment because the physical care and needs of diabetes always seem to come first.

So what can be done? First, all family members should learn about diabetes. Each should have an understanding of what it is, how to control it, and how to prevent emergencies. Also, the person with diabetes should learn to manage his or her own diabetes. Of course, the toddler with diabetes cannot be expected to take responsibility for proper diabetes control. However, as the child develops, parents should expect their son or daughter to gradually take more responsibility so that the child can learn how to control diabetes on his or her own.

Diabetes control can be stressful at times and family members should be willing to give encouragement. For example, the wife of a person with type II diabetes may want to help motivate him to exercise by being his walking or jogging partner. Or the husband of a wife with type I diabetes who is depressed over having to take insulin injections may need to spend some time to listen to her concerns and then console and assure her. Encouragement can be beneficial. However, the person with diabetes must realize that ultimately he or she is responsible for his or her own diabetes management.

Also, a person should not use diabetes to get special treatment. Of course, if you feel you have tried everything and there are still difficulties, don't hesitate to see a counselor. Diabetes can be a difficult adjustment for a family and a little professional help might be your answer. If you and your family work at it, you'll be able to conquer any challenges diabetes may pose for you.

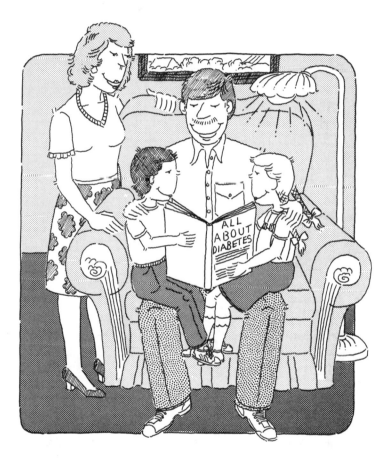

fast food
(FAST FOOD)

Having diabetes doesn't mean you are banned from Burger King or exiled from Pizza Hut. You can eat wherever you want, but you have to be choosey about what you eat. Fast foods are a lot easier than cooking at home, but with most of it, you pay a price: high calories and poor nutrition.

Because you want to keep your diabetes in control, you will want to make healthy food choices. When it comes to following proper nutritional guidelines, fast foods make the challenge even more difficult. Everyone wants to keep the calories low. The best way to do this is to buy small and eat

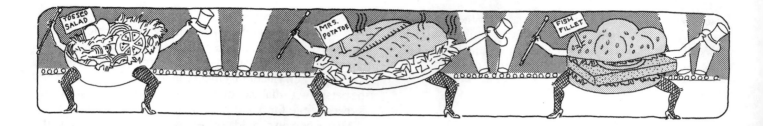

fast food facts

Product	Serving size	Calories	Carb. (gm)	Prot. (gm)	Fat (gm)	Sodium (mg)	Exchanges
ARBY'S							
Junior Roast Beef	3 oz	218	22	12	8	345	1½ Starch/Bread, 1½ Med. Fat Meat
Regular Roast Beef	5.2 oz	353	32	22	15	590	2 Starch/Bread, 2 Med. Fat Meat, 1 Fat
Hot Ham'n Cheese Sandwich	5.7 oz	353	33	26	13	1655	2 Starch/Bread, 3 Med. Fat Meat
Turkey Deluxe	7 oz	375	32	24	17	850	2 Starch/Bread, 3 Med. Fat Meat
Roasted Chicken Boneless Breast	5 oz	254	2	43	7	930	6 Lean Meat
Roasted Chicken Boneless Leg	5.35 oz	319	1	41	16	995	6 Lean Meat
Tossed Salad w/Low Calorie Italian Dressing	8 oz	57	8	3	1	465	1 Vegetable
Baked Potato, Plain	11 oz	290	66	8	1	12	4 Starch/Bread
BURGER KING							
Hamburger	1	275	29	15	12	509	2 Starch/Bread, 2 Med. Fat Meat
Cheeseburger	1	317	30	17	15	651	2 Starch/Bread, 2 Med. Fat Meat, 1 Fat
Chicken Tenders	6 pieces	204	10	20	10	636	1 Starch/Bread, 2 Med. Fat Meat
French Fries	Regular	227	24	3	13	160	1½ Starch/Bread, 2 Fat
Salad w/Reduced Italian Dressing	1	42	7	2	trace	449	1 Vegetable
BK Broiler	1	379	31	24	18	764	2 Starch, 3 Med. Fat Meat
DAIRY QUEEN							
Single Hamburger	1	360	33	21	16	630	2 Starch/Bread, 2 Med. Fat Meat, 1 Fat
Single w/cheese	1	410	33	24	20	790	2 Starch/Bread, 3 Med. Fat Meat, 1 Fat
Fish Fillet	1	430	45	20	18	674	3 Starch/Bread, 2 Med. Fat Meat, 1 Fat
French Fries	Regular	200	25	2	10	115	1½ Starch/Bread, 2 Fat
Frozen Dessert*	4 oz	180	27	4	6	65	2 Starch/Bread, 1 Fat
Cone*	Regular	240	38	6	7	80	2½ Starch/Bread, 1 Fat
Dilly Bar*	1	210	21	3	13	50	1½ Starch/Bread, 2 Fat

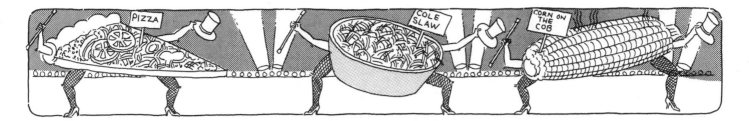

Product	Serving size	Calories	Carb. (gm)	Prot. (gm)	Fat (gm)	Sodium (mg)	Exchanges
DAIRY QUEEN (cont.)							
DQ Sandwich* *For occasional use only	1	140	24	3	4	40	1½ Starch/Bread, 1 Fat
DOMINO'S PIZZA							
Cheese Pizza 12-inch pie	2 slices	340	52	18	6	660	3 Starch/Bread, 1 Med. Fat Meat, 1 Vegetable
Pepperoni Pizza 12-inch pie	2 slices	380	48	20	12	880	3 Starch/Bread, 2 Med. Fat Meat, 1 Vegetable
HARDEE'S							
Hamburger	1 (96 gm)	276	21	14	15	589	1½ Starch/Bread, 1½ Med. Fat Meat, 1 Fat
Grilled Chicken Sandwich	1	310	34	24	9	890	2 Starch, 3 Lean Meat
Roast Beef Sandwich	1 (129 gm)	312	30	20	12	826	2 Starch/Bread, 2 Med. Fat Meat
Chef Salad	1 (336 gm)	277	10	23	16	517	2 Vegetable, 3 Med. Fat Meat
KENTUCKY FRIED CHICKEN							
Original Recipe Chicken Wing	1 (56 gm)	181	6	12	12	387	½ Starch/Bread, 1½ Med. Fat Meat, 1 Fat
Side Breast	1 (95 gm)	276	10	20	17	654	½ Starch/Bread, 3 Med. Fat Meat
Center Breast	1 (107 gm)	257	8	26	14	532	½ Starch/Bread, 3 Med. Fat Meat
Drumstick	1 (58 gm)	147	4	14	9	269	2 Med. Fat Meat
Thigh	1 (96 gm)	278	8	18	19	517	½ Starch/Bread, 2 Med. Fat Meat, 2 Fat
Kentucky Nuggets	6 (96 gm)	276	13	17	17	840	1 Starch/Bread, 2 Med. Fat Meat, 1 Fat
Hot Wings	6	376	18	22	24	677	1 Starch/Bread, 3 Med. Fat Meat, 2 Fat
Mashed Potatoes w/Gravy	1 (86 gm)	62	10	2	1	297	1 Starch/Bread
Corn-on-the-Cob	1 (143 gm)	176	32	5	3	21	2 Starch/Bread
Cole Slaw	1 (79 gm)	103	12	1	6	171	2 Vegetable or 1 Starch/Bread, 1 Fat
Baked Beans	1 (89 gm)	105	18	5	1	387	1 Starch/Bread
LONG JOHN SILVER'S							
Baked Fish Dinner w/slaw, mixed veg.	Fish w/ sauce	387	19	36	19	1298	1 Starch/Bread, 4 Med. Fat Meat
Shrimp Salad w/crackers	1	183	12	27	3	658	1 Starch/Bread, 3 Lean Meat
Ocean Chef Salad w/crackers	1	222	9	28	8	983	1 Starch/Bread, 3 Lean Meat
A La Carte: Kitchen Breaded Fish	1 (2 oz)	122	8	9	6	374	½ Starch/Bread, 1 Med. Fat Meat

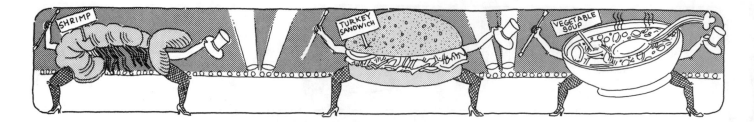

Product	Serving size	Calories	Carb. (gm)	Prot. (gm)	Fat (gm)	Sodium (mg)	Exchanges
LONG JOHN SILVER'S (cont.)							
Catfish Fillet	1 (2.7 oz)	203	13	12	12	469	1 Starch/Bread, 1 Med. Fat Meat, 1 Fat
Tender Chicken Plank	1 (2.2 oz)	152	10	9	8	515	1 Starch/Bread, 1 Med. Fat Meat
Battered Scallops	3 pc. (2.1 oz)	159	12	6	9	603	1 Starch/Bread, 1 High Fat Meat
Breaded Oysters	3 pc. (2.1 oz)	180	18	6	9	195	1 Starch/Bread, 1 High Fat Meat
Battered Shrimp	3 pc. (1.8 oz)	141	9	6	9	462	1 Starch/Bread, 1 High Fat Meat
Clam Chowder	6.6 oz	128	15	7	5	611	1 Starch/Bread, 1 Med. Fat Meat
Hushpuppies	2 pc. (1.7 oz)	145	18	3	7	405	1 Starch/Bread, 1½ Fat
McDONALD'S							
Hamburger	1 (100 gm)	263	28	12	11	506	2 Starch/Bread, 1 Med. Fat Meat, 1 Fat
Quarter Pounder	1 (160 gm)	427	29	25	23	718	2 Starch/Bread, 3 Med. Fat Meat, 1 Fat
Chicken McNuggets	6	288	17	19	16	520	1 Starch/Bread, 2 Med. Fat Meat, 1 Fat
French Fries, small	1 (68 gm)	220	26	3	12	109	2 Starch/Bread, 2 Fat
Egg McMuffin	1 (138 gm)	340	31	19	16	885	2 Starch/Bread, 2 Med. Fat Meat, 1 Fat
Scrambled Eggs	1 (98 gm)	180	2	13	13	205	2 Med. Fat Meat, 1 Fat
English Muffin w/butter	1 (63 gm)	186	30	5	5	310	2 Starch/Bread, 1 Fat
Apple Bran Muffin	1	190	46	5	0	230	3 Starch/Bread
PIZZA HUT							
Thin-n-Crispy cheese 10-inch pizza	1/2	450	54	25	15	*	3½ Starch/Bread, 2 Med. Fat Meat, 1 Fat
Thin-n-Crispy Supreme 10-inch pizza	1/2	510	51	27	21	*	3 Starch/Bread, 3 Med. Fat Meat, 1 Fat
Thick-n-Chewy Pepperoni 10-inch pizza	1/2	560	68	31	18	*	4½ Starch/Bread, 3 Med. Fat Meat
*Not available.							
RAX							
Roast Beef Sandwich	Regular	320	33	20	11	969	2 Starch/Bread, 2 Med. Fat Meat, 1 Fat
Ham & Swiss Sandwich	1 (224 gm)	430	42	23	23	1737	3 Starch/Bread, 2 Med. Fat Meat, 2 Fat
Plain Potato	1 (250 gm)	270	60	8	trace	70	4 Starch/Bread
French Fries, small	1 (3 oz)	260	33	2	13	69	2 Starch/Bread, 2 Fat
Cream of Broccoli Soup	3.5 oz	50	6	1	2	219	½ Starch/Bread
Chicken Noodle Soup	3.5 oz	40	8	2	trace	40	½ Starch/Bread

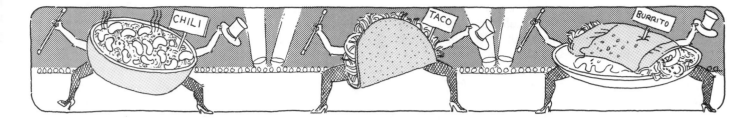

Product	Serving size	Calories	Carb. (gm)	Prot. (gm)	Fat (gm)	Sodium (mg)	Exchanges
SHAKEY'S							
Thin Cheese 13-inch pizza	1/10	140	18	9	5	315	1 Starch/Bread, 1 Med. Fat Meat
Thin Onion, Green Pepper, Olive, Mushroom 13-inch pizza	1/10	171	21	10	5	395	1 Starch/Bread, 1 Med. Fat Meat, 1 Vegetable
Thick Pepperoni 13-inch pizza	1/10	232	19	19	8	494	1 Starch/Bread, 2 Med. Fat Meat
TACO BELL							
Bean Burrito	1	343	48	11	12	272	3 Starch/Bread, 2 Fat
Beef Burrito	1	466	37	30	21	327	2½ Starch/Bread, 3 Med. Fat Meat, 1 Fat
Beef Tostada	1	291	21	19	15	138	1½ Starch/Bread, 2 Med. Fat Meat, 1 Fat
Bellbeefer	1	221	23	15	7	231	1½ Starch/Bread, 1½ Med. Fat Meat
Taco	1	186	14	15	8	79	1 Starch/Bread, 2 Lean Fat Meat
WENDY'S							
Single Hamburger Patty on white bun	1 (127 gm)	350	26	24	16	360	2 /Bread, 3 Med. Fat Meat
Plain Baked Potato	1 (250 gm)	250	52	6	2	60	3½ Starch/Bread
Chili	9 oz (256 gm)	230	16	21	9	960	1 Starch/Bread, 3 Lean Meat
Fish Fillet	1 (92 gm)	210	13	14	11	475	1 Starch/Bread, 2 Med. Fat Meat
Taco Salad	1 (791 gm)	660	46	41	37	1110	3 Starch/Bread, 5 Med. Fat Meat, 1 Fat
Pick Up Window Salad	1 (579 gm)	110	5	8	6	540	1 Vegetable, 1 Fat
Garden Spot Salad Bar:							
Lettuce, Iceberg	3 cups	20	3	trace	trace	20	1 Vegetable
Pasta Salad	¼ cup	130	18	3	6	190	1 Starch/Bread, 1 Fat
Sunflower Seeds & Raisins	1 oz	140	6	5	10	5	½ Fruit, 1 High Fat Meat
Salad Dressings: Reduced Calorie:							
Italian	2 Tbsp.	45-50	2	trace	4-5	140-180	1 Fat
ZANTIGO							
Taco	1 (84.5 gm)	198	13	10	12	318	1 Starch/Bread, 1 Med. Fat Meat, 1 Fat
Taco Burrito	1 (198.7 gm)	415	41	21	19	815	2½ Starch/Bread, 2 Med. Fat Meat, 2 Fat
Hot Cheese Chilito	1 (115.3 gm)	329	35	14	15	466	Starch/Bread, 1 Med. Fat Meat, 2 Fat

The chart is excerpted from a more extensive version in Fast Food Facts 1990 *published by the International Diabetes Center in Minneapolis. This booklet is available for $4.95 (plus postage). To order, call 1-800-848-2793.*

fasting

Fast food restaurants are getting better at offering foods low in fat, calories, and salt. Many have menus that include things such as salad bars, low-calorie salad dressings, baked potatoes, sugar-free soft drinks, and low-fat milk.

You can keep your meals low in fat by leaving off sauces such as mayonnaise and tartar sauce. Avoid foods that are deep-fried—choose broiled fish or chicken. Also, look out for processed meats like pepperoni on your pizza or sausage on your biscuit. Both are high in fat. Don't be afraid to ask that your food be prepared without extra salt.

Occasionally, eating out at your local fast food restaurant should not be a problem. Just remember to balance it out by eating well during other meals.

fasting
(FAST-ing)

Trying to lose weight by eating very little or nothing at all (fasting)? You would be better off exercising and eating less fat and calories.

Fasting can sometimes be a step toward weight loss. But unless people change their eating habits, they will gain back any weight they lose by fasting. And people with diabetes have another risk: fasting can wreak havoc on diabetes control. It is true that for some seriously overweight people with type II diabetes, a total or modified fast is sometimes used to get the weight loss started. However, those fasts are always medically supervised, usually by both a physician and a dietitian.

You may be asked to have "fasting" blood tests done. This generally means no food after midnight, if you have a morning appointment. It could also mean to go without food for 12 to 16 hours. Check with your health professional for advice.

fat exchange list
(FAT eks-CHANJ LIST)

When we say fat exchange, we are not talking about a place where you go to exchange cookie and cake recipes. Instead, these are the foods on the Fat Exchange List of the *Exchange Lists for Meal Planning*.

What are some of those things that add that ripple just above your waist? The big offenders are the saturated fats (see Fats). These include bacon, butter, and sour cream. On the unsaturated side you'll find margarine, olives, cashews, and mayonnaise. The serving sizes are small for each exchange and you're better off sticking to that amount—unless, of course, you want the fat sticking to you.

fats
(FATS)

If you're like Jack Spratt and eat no fat, you may be a step ahead of those who do. There is strong evidence that high

levels of blood fats and cholesterol increase the risk of atherosclerosis (see Atherosclerosis). And since people with diabetes are at an already increased risk for atherosclerosis, limiting your fat intake is a doubly good idea.

The good news is you can lower your blood cholesterol level and lessen the risk of atherosclerosis by changing the way you eat . . . and controlling your diabetes, of course. A general understanding of fats will help you make healthier choices at the dinner table.

There are three kinds of fats: saturated, monounsaturated, and polyunsaturated. A saturated fat is one that has been filled up (saturated) with as many hydrogen atoms as it can hold. This type of fat is usually solid at room temperature and is found mainly in animal products like lard, meat fat, and butter. Monounsaturated and polyunsaturated fats are called such because they are *not* completely saturated with hydrogen atoms—either one (mono) or many (poly) hydrogen atoms are missing. These two fats are found mainly in plant foods like oils and nuts, and are usually liquid at room temperature. The important thing to remember is that saturated fats usually raise a person's cholesterol level, while unsaturated fats tend to lower it.

Fats and cholesterol can't travel easily in the blood on their own. They attach to particles called lipoproteins (lipo means fat). Two major lipoproteins are low-density lipoproteins (LDL) and high-density lipoproteins (HDL). LDLs carry "bad cholesterol." This is because LDL can deposit its cholesterol load in the artery walls. HDL is believed to carry cholesterol away from the artery walls and back to the liver where it can be put to better use. High levels of HDL are good.

You *can* lessen the risk of atherosclerosis by altering the way you eat. If you follow your meal plan for controlling your diabetes, you are probably in great shape. But here are a few tips, in case you're interested:

■ If you are overweight, reduce the amount of calories you eat each day. Losing weight should be your top priority. It not only helps your diabetes control, it may also reduce the risk of heart disease. Check the section on weight loss for tips on losing weight.

■ Avoid eating too much saturated fat. The average American consumes two to three times more saturated fat than unsaturated fat. Ideally, you should try to balance all three fats (monounsaturated, polyunsaturated, and saturated) so that you eat equal amounts of each. It's best to limit your fat intake to 30 percent of all the calories you eat.

■ Finally, stick to your meal plan as best you can. Not only will you be able to fight atherosclerosis, but your diabetes will be in better control.

fever
(FEE-ver)

For most people, a minor fever is no big deal. But for the person with diabetes, a fever can make control difficult. For this reason, you need to take any fever seriously.

Fever is a stress and causes the body to release hormones

("stress" hormones) that raise blood sugar. This extra rise in blood glucose is meant to help the body ward off the attack.

To handle fever, you may be able to take an aspirin to lower your temperature. (Children should not take aspirin. Also, some adults should not take aspirin. Check with your doctor first.) And don't forget to drink fluids to avoid dehydration (another stress!). Also, follow the sick-day rules you have planned with your doctor. If you don't have a sick-day plan, set one up *now*—before you catch that flu on a Saturday night when your doctor is out of reach.

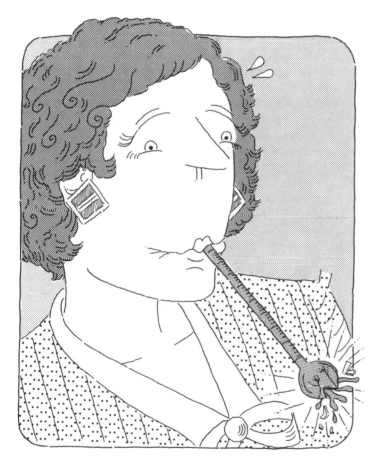

fiber
(FI-ber)

Fiber has become quite popular lately. You can hardly watch a cereal commercial without hearing the words, "high in fiber." But what is this stuff?

Fiber is found in the structural parts of plants—including the skin, roots, stems, leaves, and seeds. In reality, fiber is that part (or those parts) of plant foods that the human body cannot digest—but spends a lot of time trying to.

There are two types of fiber. One is water-soluble (breaks up in water) fiber. It is found mainly in fruits, beans, and oat products. The other is water-insoluble fiber. It is found in whole-grain breads, cereals, fruits, and vegetables.

The benefits of fiber are *still unknown*. Some studies have shown that water-soluble fiber may help control blood-glucose levels. Also, there is indication it may reduce requirements for insulin and other diabetes medication. In addition, there is evidence fiber may be helpful in reducing blood-cholesterol levels.

Both types of fiber have also been found to aid in losing weight. The water-insoluble types are bulky and take up more space in your stomach, making you feel full. This means you'll probably eat less. The water-soluble takes longer to exit the stomach, so you feel full longer.

While not all is known about fiber, we do know it is beneficial and nutritionists have recommended increasing your fiber intake. If you look at the American Diabetes Association's *Exchange Lists for Meal Planning*, you will notice a wheat stalk by some foods to help you identify those high in fiber.

While there are benefits to fiber, some precautions should be noted:
■ Check with your doctor before increasing the amount of fiber in your diet, particularly if you have autonomic neuropathy (nerve damage caused by long-standing diabetes—see Neuropathy).
■ Increase your fiber intake by choosing *natural* foods in their original casings. Good examples are brown rice, dried beans, peas, and lentils.
■ Avoid purified fiber supplements.
■ Do not take high-fiber foods in addition to the carbohydrates already in your diet.

finding a dietitian
(FIN-ding A DI-a-TISH-an)

A dietitian is a valuable member on your health-care team. Because good nutrition counseling is far more than a printed meal plan, you will want to find a dietitian who you can work with and can help design meal plans that will meet your needs. With information about your lifestyle and medical needs, you and your dietitian will be able to set up an individualized meal plan that will give you a variety of meals to choose from. And from time to time, you will want to meet to discuss how you are adapting to your new eating patterns, and how well they are working for you.

Of course, before you do all that, you need to choose a dietitian. First, look for one that is a registered dietitian (R.D.). Your doctor may be able to recommend one. Some hospital outpatient clinics offer nutrition counseling for people with diabetes. Or, check with your American Diabetes Association chapter or affiliate.

After you get a few names to choose from, call them and get a feeling for how they work. Ask whether you will be given an individualized meal plan. What information will the dietitian want from you? Good dietitians will want to know your medical history, as well as things like food allergies and food preferences.

Once you have found a good dietitian, be prepared to keep a diary of what you eat for a few days. Be honest about your food likes and dislikes and your diary. As you and your dieti-

finding a pharmacist

tian work together, you should be able to construct a meal plan that will meet your tastes and help you keep your diabetes in control.

If you find you stray from your meal plan often, there may be something wrong with the plan. Your dietitian should work with you as your needs change—both to fit your medical and personal needs. Your dietitian should also be able to help you design a meal plan for such things as weight loss or special occasions. Finally, check your insurance plan—it may cover your visits with the dietitian.

finding a pharmacist
(FIN-ding A FAR-ma-sist)

Some people consider pharmacists to be mere sellers of medicines. These people have no personal interaction with their pharmacist. That can be a great mistake. A quality pharmacist can provide services far beyond the sale of drugs.

Look for a pharmacist who keeps a patient profile, a written record of drugs you have used, special diets, prescribed therapy, and chronic illnesses like diabetes, hypertension, or heart disease. This can then be used to monitor your therapy, prevent you from using two drugs that do not mix well together, and alert you to drugs or food that might interfere with control.

Good pharmacists also will give you advice on storing drugs, saving money by buying generic drugs (when possible), and how to take prescription and over-the-counter drugs. Your pharmacist can also warn you about products containing alcohol or sugar, which can affect blood-glucose levels.

Your local American Diabetes Association affiliate may be able to supply names of pharmacists interested in diabetes. Other good sources of information are your physician and friends. Remember, you spend a lot of money in your pharmacy and are entitled to the best possible service. Take advantage of your pharmacist's knowledge.

finding a physician
(FIN-ding A fi-ZISH-un)

Your physician is not just there to give diagnoses, prescribe treatments, and monitor your condition. Your doctor can also be a valuable resource when you have other health care needs, such as choosing a dietitian or a diabetes educational program. As a cornerstone in your quality of life, your physician should be chosen with care.

How do you find a doctor? You may want to first try your local American Diabetes Association affiliate or chapter to see if they have a listing of doctors in your area who specialize in diabetes or have a special interest in persons with diabetes. Many hospitals also have lists of doctors to choose from. Neighbors or friends may also be able to give you names of doctors that have a good reputation.

Once you have the names of doctors to choose from, you will want to check them out to see if they will meet your needs. Don't be afraid to shop around for a doctor. *You* are the health-care consumer. If you are not happy with your doctor, you won't seek care when it is needed and may not follow medical recommendations—and that can be hazardous to your health.

One thing to look for is a doctor who shows a keen interest in diabetes and is current on the latest research. Of course, you will want a doctor who is qualified, but qualifications are

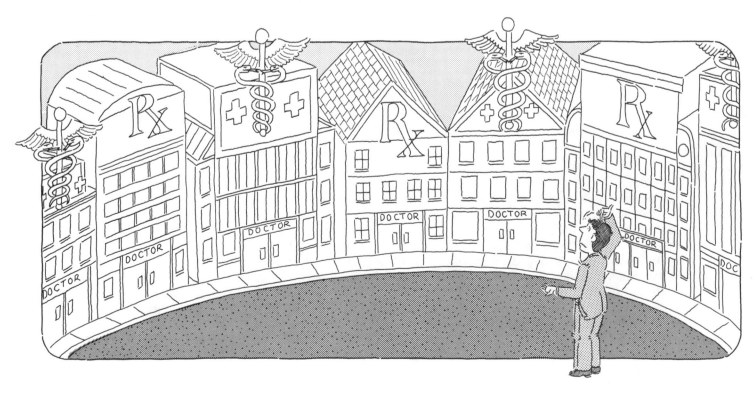

not enough. You and your doctor must be relaxed and able to talk freely together and should respect and trust one another. You may be able to get a feel for your doctor by being aware of the atmosphere on your first visit. Do you feel comfortable with the office staff? With the physician? Were you rushed when you tried to ask questions? Were your questions answered?

Also during that first visit, find out such things as what hospital the doctor is affiliated with, how often your visits should be, and how you can reach the doctor in an emergency. The more information you can find out, the easier it will be to choose a doctor.

When you finally find the doctor you like, have your previous physician send your medical records to your new doctor, so the most complete history is available.

Finally, don't feel you are stuck with a doctor, even after several visits. If you're not happy with the doctor you choose, discuss your concerns with the doctor. If your concerns are not resolved, look for another doctor who better meets your needs. Your health is all-important and one of the keys to good health is being happy. And if you're not happy with your doctor, you won't be healthy.

finding a podiatrist
(FIN-ding A po-DI-a-trist)

See Foot Care

finding a psychotherapist
(FIN-ding A si-KO-THER-a-pist)

Diabetes isn't all in the body. Your feelings can affect your diabetes control, and your diabetes can affect your feelings. You may need help in accepting and coping with the burdens and challenges of diabetes. Or you may need help in coping with the stresses of life—which, on top of everything else, can throw your diabetes out of control. Therapists (psychologists, psychiatrists, etc.) are professionals trained to help you do all these things.

Your physician may have a recommendation, or your local American Diabetes Association affiliate may be able to give you the names of therapists with a special interest in diabetes. In addition, family service organizations and clinics often offer low-cost counseling. Find these services in the *Yellow Pages* under such listings as "Mental Health Services" and "Clinics."

If coping with stress is your concern, you also might check with the local "Y" continuing education programs, or the psychology department at a nearby university.

Many people are willing to accept help for physical problems, but run from the thought of seeking help for emotional ones. That's a shame—and doubly so if you let emotional problems get in the way of good diabetes management.

food labels
(FOOD LA-bels)

Have you ever sat down and read a food label? No? Well, you might want to consider it—that is, if you want to keep your diabetes in control.

What does reading food labels have to do with maintaining diabetes control? A lot. If you know what is in the food contained in that tin can, plastic wrapper, or cardboard box, you can better determine whether or not that food fits your healthy meal plan. We have some information that should help you unscramble the ingredients code.

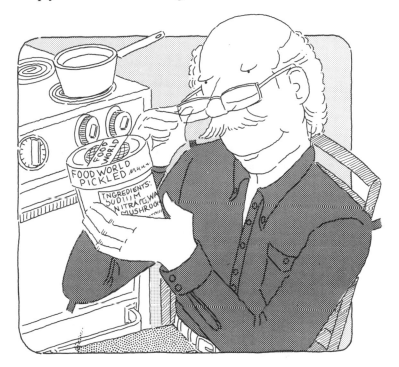

First, look at a list of ingredients on some food package you have in your home. These ingredients are listed in order according to their weight. The one with the most weight is listed first. For example, if you see that sugar is listed first and salt listed seventh, this means there is more sugar by weight than salt.

You will want to keep an eye out for sugars. But that may not be as easy as it sounds since there are a variety of names for sugars. Here are a few you may see listed on food packages: sucrose, fructose, dextrose, maltose, high-fructose corn syrup, cane sugar, invert sugar, molasses, honey, cane sweetener, fruit sugar, brown sugar, and raw sugar. New sugars come on the market occasionally. Your dietitian or doctor can keep you up to date on these new sugars.

The same is true of salt. When a label lists monosodium glutamate, sodium citrate, sodium hydroxide, sodium propionate, baking powder, baking soda, or sodium nitrate, the product has salt. You need to avoid foods with those ingredients if you are on a salt-restricted diet.

Now, let's look at the nutrition label. Government regulations require makers of food products to list serving sizes. The serving sizes must be listed in common measurements like

food labels

teaspoons, ounces, cups, or even pieces. The label also lists the calories per serving and the weight of protein, carbohydrates, and fats *in grams per serving*. For example, one can of vegetables may be listed as 1¾ servings; the nutrient labeling is for one serving only—*not* for the entire can. There must be a listing of the percentages of United States Recommended Daily Allowances of vitamins A and C and other nutrients. One thing you need to remember, however, is that the serving sizes are determined by the manufacturer—the serving sizes may not equal yours.

Then how can you figure packaged foods into your food exchanges? The printed chart below is a start. Below are some

calculating exchanges from food labels

Step 1: List the main ingredients and determine which Exchange Groups they fall into.

Step 2: From the package, list the grams of carbohydrate, protein, and fat in 1 **suggested serving** List the calories, too.

Step 3: Figure out, and then list, the number of exchanges in the most prominent Exchange Group, in this case, Starch/Bread. To find the number of Starch/Bread Exchanges, divide the number of carbohydrate grams in one serving (32 grams) by the number of carbohydrate grams in 1 **exchange** (15 grams). You can use the carbohydrate because that's the main component of Starch/Bread exchanges. (32g. divided by 15g. = 2 $\frac{2}{15}$ Starch/Bread, which rounds off to 2 Starch/Bread Exchanges.) If 1 Starch/Bread Exchange has 15 grams of carbohydrate, 3 grams of protein, a trace of fat, and 80 calories, then 2 Starch/Bread Exchanges have 30 grams of carbohydrate (2 x 15g.), 6 grams of protein (2 x 3g.) and 160 calories (2 x 80 cal.)

Step 4: Subtract the amounts of carbohydrate, protein, fat, and calories you get in Step 3 from the amounts listed on the label to see how much of each would be "left over."

Step 5: Go to the next major Exchange Group in Step 1 and repeat Steps 3 and 4 until almost no carbohydrate, protein, fat, and calories remain. The next food group here is High-Fat Meat, which is a protein list. To see how many exchanges you have, divide the **remaining protein** (4 grams) by the amount of protein in 1 **exchange** (7 grams). (4g. divided by 7g. = ⁴⁄₇ Meats, or 1 High-Fat Meat Exchange.) From the table, you know that 1 High-Fat Meat has 7 grams of protein, 8 grams of fat, and 100 calories.

Step 6: List Exchanges for 1 serving.

Main Ingredients		Exchange Groups		
Macaroni Chedder Cheese		Starch/Bread High-Fat Meat		
Serving	Carb. (g.)	Pro. (g.)	Fat	Cal.
¾ cup	32	10	7	240
2 Starch/Bread	30	6	—	160
(Results of subtracting	2	4	7	80
1 High-Fat Meat (results of subtracting)	—	7	8	100
	2	−3	−1	−20

¾ cup = 2 Starch/Bread Exchange and 1 High-Fat Meat Exchange additional comments that may help you figure your exchanges from packaged food:

■ If a food is mostly *carbohydrate* (bread, cereal, pasta, flour, or starchy vegetables), you will generally start your calculations by determining the type of exchange such as the Starch/Bread exchanges. If the food is mostly sugar, start with the Fruit exchanges. If it's mostly protein, start with Meat exchanges; mostly milk, start with Milk exchanges; mostly fat, start with Fat exchanges.

■ As a rule, round off fractions. Drop exchanges that are less than half. If the exchange is more than half, round up and count the exchange as one. If the exchange is exactly half, count it as half of an exchange.

■ Be aware that foods may not fit into your exchange groups exactly. Don't worry if you have two to three grams of carbohydrate, protein, or fat left over. But do not vary from your *daily* meal plan by more than five grams in any category or by more than 40 calories.

foot care
(FOOT KARE)

How would you like to be a foot—stuffed into sweaty socks and cramped shoes, pounded against concrete, being stepped on at times?

OK, you are not a foot. But you do have feet and you do have diabetes. The two go together, you know—both need constant care so you can lead a normal, healthy, and happy life. Because you have diabetes, you need to take special care of your feet. If circulation is poor or nerve impulses are impaired (neuropathy) in your feet, you should be especially concerned. Poor circulation prevents foot tissues from fighting infections. These infections could lead to gangrene (see Gangrene and Amputation). Impaired nerves may keep you from feeling pain and realizing that your feet need attention.

Want some tips on how to care for your feet? Great! Here they are:

■ Have your feet checked by a doctor at least once a year.

■ Wash your feet daily and dry them carefully, especially between the toes.

■ Check your feet daily for redness, blisters, cuts or scratches, cracks between the toes, discoloration, or irritation. Treat irritations only with antiseptics recommended by your doctor. If an infection occurs, report it immediately to your doctor or podiatrist.

■ Steer clear of corn plasters or commercial corn cures. These preparations destroy skin tissue, leaving your feet open to infections and calluses.

■ Guard against cuts and irritations. Put a light on when you walk around your home at night and never go barefoot.

■ Wear properly fitted shoes. They should fit well when you buy them. But even the best-fitting shoes should be worn only for short periods at a time at first. Before putting on shoes, check them for pebbles, torn linings, protruding nails, and the like.

■ Cut your nails straight across above the toeline. Let your doctor take care of hangnails.

■ Be careful of burns, including sunburns. Do not use hot water bottles and heating pads. Stay out of water that seems too hot. In all these cases, if you have any loss of sensation, you can burn your feet without realizing it.

■ Socks or nylons should be even and smooth. Socks that are mended or bumpy can put extra pressure on your feet. Change your socks every day.

■ Avoid doing things that restrict blood flow to your feet. Smoking is one. It can lead to narrowed blood vessels. Other things that can restrict blood flow are crossing your legs, exposing your feet to the cold, or wearing elastic garters or socks with tight elastic tops.

Did you get all of that? You may want to *walk* through these *steps* again to get a *foot*hold on proper foot care. Excuse the puns, but don't excuse proper foot care.

free foods
(FREE FOODS)

It may be true that there is no such thing as a free lunch, but there are such things as free foods—at least when it comes to meal planning. Free foods are "free" because you can eat as much as you want of those foods on the list that have no specific serving size. Some items on the list (such as sugar-free pancake syrup and low-calorie salad dressing) have serving sizes and you are limited to a specific number of servings per day for these items.

Some of the free foods without any serving size are: lettuce; spinach; celery; zucchini; hard, sugar-free candy; unsweetened dill pickles; black coffee and tea; club soda; and sugar-free gum. Some of the foods with serving sizes are: unsweetened cranberries and rhubarb (1/2 cup), whipped topping (2 Tbsp.), and sugar-free jam or jelly (2 Tsp.). Also included among the free foods are the seasonings—everything from basil to Worcestershire sauce.

We've given you a "taste" of the free foods list contained in the *Exchange Lists for Meal Planning*. If you would like a copy of the booklet that lists all the exchanges, including the free foods, contact your local American Diabetes Association affiliate or chapter.

fruit exchange list
(FROOT eks-CHANJ LIST)

Take your pick—an apple, an orange, a kiwi, a pear; blackberries, blueberries, cherries, and figs—all exist on the Fruit Exchange list.

Of course, you have to be careful to get the right amount to fit your meal plan. To do this, you need to be aware of what an exchange is. For example, before you peel down the skin on a banana, understand that one exchange equals only half a banana. But you can have two medium-sized persimmons for one exchange. Or you can eat three whole prunes, if you

gangrene

dare. If you can't find your favorite fruit on the list, a basic rule to follow is one exchange equals a ½ cup of fresh fruit or fruit juice. Measure ¼ cup for dried fruit.

We hope you had a peachy time reading this bit of information. Now, orange you glad you read it?

gangrene
(GANG-green)

It's a shame—in fact, an outrage—that people with diabetes are still losing limbs to gangrene, because gangrene is often *preventable*.

Gangrene happens when the blood supply to a tissue is cut off for six hours or more. The tissue becomes numb and dark-colored and dies. Dead tissue must be amputated. Unfortunately, amputation of seemingly good tissue is often necessary to save the rest of the limb.

Many times gangrene sets in after a person cuts a foot but doesn't realize it, possibly because neuropathy (nerve damage) prevents the person from feeling pain. Left untreated, the cut becomes infected and then severely infected. If circulation in the foot is bad, the chances for infection are high. Regular blood flow helps to nourish tissues and heal infections; on the other hand, weak circulation promotes infection because too few healing agents reach the affected area. If the infection becomes severe enough, the damaged tissues die and gangrene sets in. (There is also a form of gangrene, known as "dry gangrene," that is caused by poor circulation alone. This happens when an artery or arteries become blocked. Because the blood is unable to reach and nourish the area that is blocked, tissue dies.)

The keys to preventing gangrene are: Check your feet every night; be alert to any blisters, discoloration, infections or any other changes to your feet; and see your doctor or podiatrist as soon as any of these signs appear. (More detailed instructions are outlined in the section titled Foot Care.) The way to keep a foot problem minor is to report it while it is still minor. You *are not* wasting your doctor's time!

generic drugs
(jah-NARE-ik DRUGS)

Have you ever taken acetaminophen? Well, you may not have been aware of it, but you may have taken it to relieve your headache. Acetaminophen is the *generic* name for Tylenol.

What is a generic drug? When a drug is invented it is given two names. The first one is the generic, or chemical, name that describes what it is. The other one is the brand name, the one the manufacturer uses to market the drug.

When a company first develops a drug, it takes out a patent on the drug's chemical composition. For 17 years no other company can sell that drug. After the 17 years, other companies may choose to sell the drug under the generic name

or will come up with their own "brand" name. These companies cannot sell their version of the drug without receiving approval from the Food and Drug Administration.

Why settle for the generic when you can get the original? Because the generic drugs are generally cheaper. But cheaper may not mean a better deal. These drugs may not be identical to the brand name original. The rates at which they are absorbed into the body may differ. This may not be critical if you're trying to cure a headache, but may be if you are taking a glucose-lowering drug. Oral agents that are absorbed too quickly can lower blood sugar too quickly. Ones that work too slowly may not curb high blood sugar.

If you are thinking about switching to a generic, these words of advice will come in handy:

■ Before switching to a generic drug, talk to your doctor. Some doctors advise care when switching from one drug to another—particularly once your body has gotten used to one certain drug. If you do switch, make sure you and your doctor monitor your reactions in case your body reacts differently to the new drug.

■ Ask your pharmacist to inform you if there is a change in the manufacturer of the drug you are using. The quality and absorption rates may change.

■ Take all medications according to your doctor's and pharmacist's instructions.

genetic links
(jah-NET-ik LINKS)

The search for genetic roots to diabetes is a true detective story. Researchers have long known that both type I and type II diabetes tend to run in families—although having a relative with diabetes does not guarantee that you will develop it. But pinpointing the specific genes that put a person at risk for developing diabetes has been a puzzle. (Genes are microscopic biochemical units that determine a person's hereditary traits, such as color of hair and eyes, and height.) Scientists are trying to track down these genes by studying substances called HLAs. (HLA stands for Human Leukocyte Antigen.)

HLAs are proteins that sit on the surfaces of many cells, including the beta cells of the pancreas (the insulin-producers). These antigens play a role in the body's defense (immune) system. There are different kinds of HLAs so people can have them in different combinations. Your particular combination is determined by your genes. But having the "right" genes isn't enough to bring on diabetes. Investigators know that something in the environment triggers the process that turns on diabetes. That something can be a virus, such as the flu or pneumonia (in the case of type I), or obesity or a poor diet (in the case of type II).

Among people with type I diabetes, investigators have found that several particular HLAs turn up repeatedly. So these HLAs may eventually be used one day to more precisely predict a given individual's risk of developing type I diabetes.

But this does not mean a person with these HLAs will necessarily develop diabetes. What it does mean is a person with certain HLAs is more susceptible to developing diabetes. And from what researchers currently understand, some who do not have these certain HLAs may even develop diabetes.

Unfortunately, scientists don't fully understand how these antigens relate to type II diabetes. Researchers know that someone in a family with a history of type II diabetes is at higher risk of developing the disease than others with no such history. They also know that where type I diabetes is rare and often seems to come from nowhere, type II diabetes is

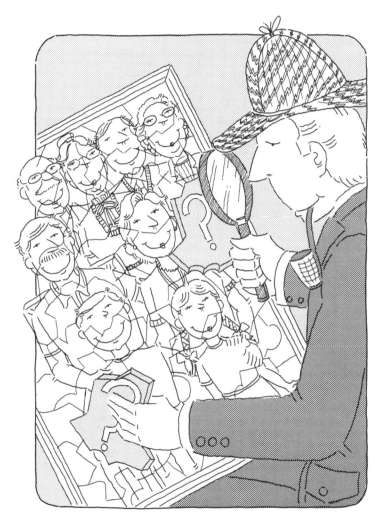

"handed down" from generation to generation. But the specific genes are still a mystery. (Sometimes, eating habits and lifestyle that can lead to type II are also handed down.)

Scientists have much to learn before they understand the role that heredity plays—along with other important factors, such as viruses and obesity—in the development of diabetes. But the hope is that with greater understanding, physicians may eventually be able to intervene to prevent type I and type II diabetes in high-risk individuals.

gestational diabetes
(jes-TA-shun-al DI-a-BEET-eez)

This type of diabetes is developed by some women during pregnancy. Usually, gestational diabetes disappears after the baby is born. However, nearly 50 percent of these women will eventually develop type II diabetes.

What does pregnancy have to do with women getting diabetes? During the last few months of pregnancy, the placenta secretes hormones that can raise the mother's blood-glucose levels. (The placenta is the "sack" in which the baby develops.) Women who cannot produce enough insulin to match the glucose in the blood may be diagnosed as having gestational diabetes.

If diabetes during pregnancy is not well controlled, the woman risks having an extremely large baby. This is because the mother's excess glucose passes through the placenta to the baby. The baby uses the extra glucose from the mother's blood and grows large and chubby. The size of the baby can put the pregnancy at risk. In addition, because these babies are processing both their own and their mother's glucose, they must be closely monitored for the first several hours after birth to make certain they do not suffer from hypoglycemia (low blood sugar).

Nowadays, all women should be checked for the development of diabetes during pregnancy. If you have gestational diabetes, your doctor will want you to treat it carefully. Expect to follow a carefully controlled meal plan. You may even need to take insulin. Maintaining normal blood-glucose levels will be important. Also, after the baby is born, you will want to watch for signs of diabetes (excessive thirst, frequent urination, irritability, nausea, hunger—see Diabetes) and have periodic checkups.

Women who have a family history of diabetes, are older than 30, or have delivered stillborn, overweight infants should also be checked for diabetes before becoming pregnant.

glucagon
(GLOO-kah-gone)

Glucagon is a hormone that raises blood sugar. It is used primarily as a medication to treat someone with diabetes who has passed out from a severe insulin reaction. (See Hypoglycemia.)

Glucagon is only available by prescription. Ask your doctor to prescribe it for you (especially if you have difficulty recognizing the warning signs of an insulin reaction, and preventing a reaction from happening). And ask your doctor to discuss how and when to use glucagon. Glucagon is injected the same way as insulin and usually takes effect in about 15 or 20 minutes. As soon as the person is able, he or she should cat something with sugar in it until he or she is alert. If the individual fails to come out of the insulin reaction, call the paramedics or take the person to the hospital.

glycosylated hemoglobin

(Attempts should be made to discover what caused the insulin reaction, so that further reactions can be prevented.)

Be sure that family members and co-workers know how to give you a glucagon injection, should you ever need it. Being prepared for such emergencies is part of properly managing your diabetes.

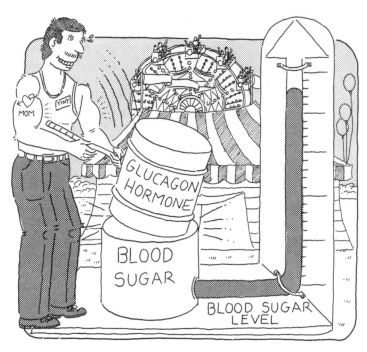

glycosylated hemoglobin
(gli-KOS-eh-late-ed HE-mo-GLOW-bin)

Glycosylated hemoglobin, glycohemoglobin, or hemoglobin A_{1C} (pronounced A-one-C)—all hard-to-pronounce terms for a very important test.

This test, which is ordered by your doctor, measures the average control of your diabetes four to eight weeks prior to the test. Here's how: When blood-glucose levels are high, some of the glucose attaches to hemoglobin molecules in red blood cells. The glucose stays attached for the remaining life of the hemoglobin cell. (These cells live about 120 days.) Through this test, your doctor is able to see your pattern of control during the past one to two months. The results from this test can help you and your doctor adjust your diet and insulin to improve diabetes control.

hands
(HANDS)

Do your hands hurt you? We don't quite understand the reasons, but people with long-standing diabetes are more susceptible to four kinds of hand problems. What doctors do know is that the disorders are easy to diagnose and relatively easy to correct. If you have any of the following symptoms,

talk them over with your doctor:

■ Carpal Tunnel Syndrome. Symptoms are burning, tingling, or numbness, usually in the thumb, index, third, and part of the fourth fingers. These symptoms may get worse at night. The pain is caused by pressure on a nerve that runs through the wrist to the hand. The pressure occurs when a ligament in the wrist becomes inflamed and swollen. The condition can be made worse by activities involving repeated wrist motion, such as wringing clothes.

The pain generally can be eased by tilting the hand backward slightly at the wrist to relieve the pressure. One treatment is to wear a splint, mainly at night, to keep the hand in this position. Sometimes a steroid injection into the ligament is given to reduce inflammation. If you have this done, your diabetes control must be monitored carefully because steroids can raise blood glucose. If neither method helps, surgery may be necessary.

■ "Trigger Finger." The technical name for this is "stenosing tenosynovitis." It usually affects the middle or ring finger, causing it to thicken. That finger will hurt when moved and will eventually lock in a bent position. Again, the cause is swollen tissues, this time in the tendons of the fingers. Surgery may be necessary to release the locked finger by removing the scar tissue that binds the tendon.

■ Limited Joint Mobility (LJM). LJM is painless and may slightly limit flexibility of some joints, such as those in the hands and feet. LJM may not cause you much discomfort or limit your ability to perform daily tasks. However, diagnosing LJM is important, because it may alert the doctor to the presence of microvascular complications (those involving small blood vessels) common in people with diabetes, such as retinopathy (eye disease). During your regular check-up, your doctor may check for signs of LJM by shaking both your hands; this is done to check for any stiffness of the skin. To check for flexibility, he or she may then ask you to put your palms together in a clapping or "prayer" position, with your forearms parallel to the floor. While your palms are touching, your doctor may then ask you to pull your fingers back away from the fingers on the other hand. If your doctor does diagnose LJM, he or she may have you tested for retinopathy or other microvascular complications.

■ Dupuytren's Contracture. This disorder affects the palm and fingers, usually not with real pain, but more often a dull ache, tingling, numbness, or stiffness. For some reason, scar tissue develops in the sheath around the muscles and other tissue in the palm. This is the start. Then, bumps may appear and, eventually, the palm may become thick, hard, and dimpled. Sometimes the fingers bend into the palm. All this occurs over the course of years. Fortunately, in severe cases, surgery can help restore movement.

health-care team
(HELTH-KARE TEEM)

It is important to manage your diabetes properly so that you can live a healthy and full life. Good management requires the help of your health-care team. Your team should consist of professionals who know your needs, can set and make adjustments for controlling your diabetes (exercise, meal planning, and insulin and/or pills), and can spot problems that may accompany diabetes early before they become serious.

A typical team should include your doctor, a dietitian, a diabetes nurse-educator, and other professionals you may need, such as an eye doctor, a podiatrist (foot specialist), and possibly a psychologist or social worker. Remember, this team should be on your side—they should be concerned about your well-being and be willing to answer any questions you have. They should also be able to help you make adjustments in managing your diabetes to fit changes in your lifestyle.

And don't forget, you are part of this team, which means doing *your* part by following the guidelines to keep your diabetes in control. The more you and your health-care team work together, the better the chances your diabetes control will be a winner.

health maintenance organizations

(HELTH MAIN-ten-ans OR-ga-ni-ZA-shuns)

It's easier to call them HMOs and it may prove to be an easier and less expensive way for you to receive health care.

Health maintenance organizations offer a change from the traditional fee-for-service health plans most of us are used to. In a fee-for-service type plan, you and/or your employer pay a premium (a fixed monthly fee), plus you agree to pay a percentage of the cost (called a copayment). Also, you usually have to meet a deductible. (A deductible is the amount you agree to pay before your insurance begins coverage. If your deductible is $500, your insurance will not pay anything until your total bills exceed $500).

An HMO works differently. In an HMO, you and/or your employer pay a fixed fee (usually monthly) for a wide range of medical services. You usually do not pay anything more than that fixed fee.

The services you can receive will range from routine office visits to hospitalization. Be sure to check what an HMO will cover before signing up. Like many insurance policies, the HMO may not cover your complete medical needs. For example, an HMO may not cover the costs of diabetes education or testing supplies. The HMO may only offer limited coverage for these services. Shop around to see that you find the best HMO for you.

Unlike the traditional fee-for-service plans, an HMO may be limited in giving you a choice of doctors and hospitals. Some HMOs only allow you to receive services from the doctors on the HMO staff and from hospitals under contract with the HMO. If you like a particular doctor or hospital and they are not connected to the HMO, you may be out of luck. But, HMOs will usually cover the costs of a hospital or doctor used during an emergency. For example, if you are out of town, need medical attention and are in an area not covered by your HMO, your HMO will probably cover you. Also, some HMOs may not have the specialist you need. However, many HMOs will cover the cost of a specialist if they cannot provide one.

There are advantages and disadvantages to HMOs. You are more likely to get the regular checkups you need because there is no extra cost. In fact, most HMOs encourage checkups to head off problems before they get worse. However, if you have diabetes, a fee-for-service plan may be a better choice because it may pay for routine diabetes checkups.

HMOs do offer convenience. You don't have to fill out forms or file claims. Most of your services will be paid. And you won't have to worry about out-of-pocket expenses should a serious, unexpected illness come along.

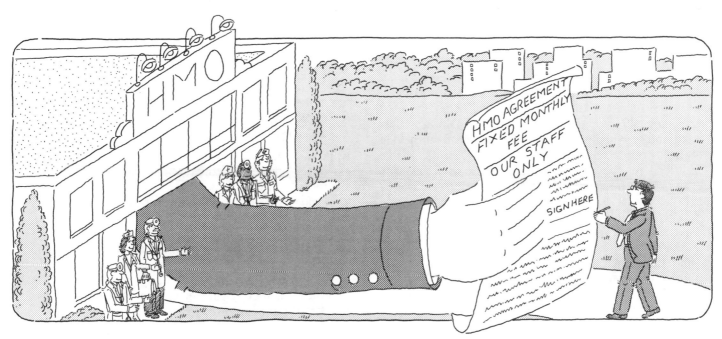

heart

heart

(HART)

To call it a "pump" somehow doesn't do it justice. No pump you can buy will keep running continuously for decades, never stopping for a breather or an occasional spare part. Yet this is exactly the performance we want—and by and large *get*—from our hearts.

Unfortunately the heart does not always perform as we would like it to. Heart disease, mainly *coronary* artery disease, occurs often enough—or severely enough—to be the leading cause of death in the United States. And, for reasons still poorly understood, the risk is higher for those with diabetes than those without.

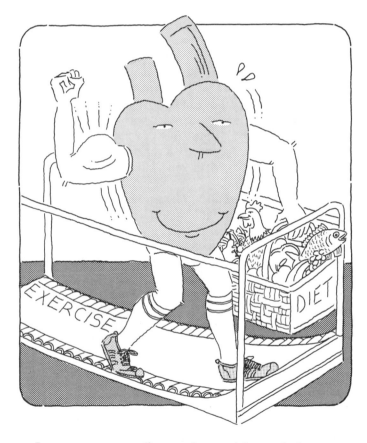

In coronary artery disease, the special vessels (coronary arteries) that feed the heart muscle become blocked or narrowed (see Atherosclerosis). This blockage stops the heart from getting all the nourishment it needs and the heart may lose its ability to pump blood efficiently (heart failure). Pain (angina)—often described as a crushing, pressure-like sensation—may develop in the chest, neck, and arms, and eventually, the heart muscle itself may become damaged or die (a heart attack).

Diabetes is only one of a number of factors linked to a higher risk of coronary artery disease. Others include:
- smoking
- high blood pressure
- high levels of fats and cholestrol (a fat-like substance) in the blood
- a family history of *premature* (before the age of 55-60)

heart disease
- lack of exercise
- obesity

Many of these factors (particularly smoking) are under your direct control. So, the way you take care of yourself, and how you work with your physician, plays a large role in your heart's health.

The main warning signs of coronary disease are:
- chest pain. This sometimes occurs after a period of exercise or a heavy meal.
- shortness of breath (greater than you might expect if you're out of shape, or it is waking you in the night)
- sweating, dizziness, nausea
- swollen ankles. This may be a sign your heart is not pumping properly.
- irregular heart beat

Report any of these signs to your doctor immediately. And have regular checkups. Your doctor can check important signs such as blood pressure and heart rate. If heart problems are suspected, your doctor may refer you to a cardiologist (heart specialist) for extra testing.

Heart ailments—the most common of which is high blood pressure—are often treated with medicines. Most medications have only minor effects on your diabetes control, but some—such as propanolol (Inderal) and many diuretics—can upset your blood-glucose level. Be sure that the doctor treating your heart knows you have diabetes.

There have been some exciting advances in heart surgery. One is coronary bypass procedures. In a bypass, a natural or artificial length of blood vessel is used to create a detour around a blocked portion of an artery. When all goes well, normal blood flow is restored.

Another procedure is called angioplasty or *balloon dilatation*. In this technique, a long, thin balloon is inserted into a blocked artery. When inflated, the balloon packs excess fat, cholesterol, and other material against the vessel wall. This procedure allows more blood to flow through the artery. The technique, which can only be performed on large blood vessels only, is less risky than full-scale surgery, but its long-term effectiveness is uncertain.

Diabetes alone does not make a person a poor candidate for either of these procedures. However, if a person has widespread blockages in the small blood vessels, clearing large blood vessels may not accomplish much. Some researchers believe that diabetes contributes to blood-vessel blockages.

How can you help prevent heart problems?

- First, keep your diabetes under control. High blood glucose is one suspected cause of heart and blood-vessel disorders.
- Second, *don't smoke*. Smoking is one of the major causes of atherosclerosis both in the heart and in other parts of the body.
- Keep high blood pressure under control. You can do this by limiting your salt intake and taking prescribed medication.
- Finally, eating properly especially to try to lower blood cholesterol, and exercising regularly are two things that will help keep your heart problems in check.

Does this advice sound familiar? If it doesn't, turn to the section titled *Control* and start learning how to take care of your diabetes and your heart as well.

heat wave
(HEET WAVE)

Ever been out on a blistering-hot day and thought you were going to drop? If you were not careful and suffered from heat exhaustion, or worse, heat stroke, you just might have.

Heat exhaustion occurs when your body loses excessive salt and water when you perspire. Symptoms include paleness, excessive sweating, nausea, and possibly, vomiting. If you suffer from heat exhaustion you should rest in a cool place. You should also drink lots of fluids and eat foods that go along with your meal plan. As soon as possible, you should be taken to the hospital to have fluid replaced into your body.

Heat stroke, which is more serious, happens when your body cannot cool itself down. One of the first signs of heat stroke is feeling lethargic. More severe signs are having a fever above 103 degrees F, being in a coma or a semi-comatose state, and dry skin. A person with heat stroke should be kept cool and taken immediately to a hospital.

Those especially at risk to heat emergencies include the elderly, people who use diuretics (pills that help rid the body of fluids), and people with diabetes. High blood glucose can lead to dehydration (water loss), which can put a person at risk for heat disorders. Some precautions to take on hot days:

■ Keep diabetes in control.
■ Avoid strenuous exercise during the hottest times of the

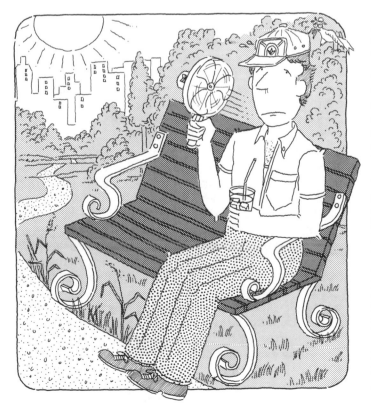

day. Save that jogging stint for early in the morning or late in the evening. And don't be active in the heat at all unless you've adapted to the temperature gradually. (Travelers to hot climates take note!)

■ Drink enough liquid. If you tend to perspire a lot, ask your doctor which liquids will help you replace salt and find out whether these beverages are safe for you. People with high blood pressure, for example, have to limit salt.
■ Stay out of direct sunlight as much as possible.
■ Invest in air conditioning. If you are elderly and have a low income, check with the electric company in early spring about possible financial arrangements.
■ Do whatever you can to keep cool. Bathe, shower, sponge yourself with cool water, and wear wide-brimmed hats and loose cotton clothes. You may also want to carry an umbrella to keep the sun off you.

high blood pressure
(HI BLUD PRESH-er)

The medical term is hypertension, but this condition does not necessarily mean a person is tense. High blood pressure occurs when blood pushes too hard against the walls of the blood vessels. It should be taken seriously because of the damage it can cause throughout the body, particularly in major organs such as the heart, kidneys, eyes, and brain.

Hypertension occurs more frequently in people who have diabetes than among those who don't. But diabetes may not be the direct cause—other factors may contribute, such as diet and excess weight. In fact, in most cases the precise cause of high blood pressure remains unknown.

People with diabetes must control hypertension because many of the complications of high blood pressure are similar or identical to those of diabetes. Both hypertension and diabetes can contribute to atherosclerosis (see Atherosclerosis). And atherosclerosis, in turn, can cause peripheral vascular disease (impaired blood flow, especially in the legs) and heart disease. In addition, hypertension can aggravate kidney disease, a common complication from long-standing diabetes. So diabetes and hypertension can put you at high risk for life-threatening problems.

Can you spot high blood pressure coming? Hypertension usually has no outward symptoms—thus its nickname, the silent killer. That's why it is important to have your blood pressure checked regularly. You can have it checked during your regular checkup with your doctor. Your doctor may want you to have it checked more often.

Fortunately, high blood pressure can be controlled. Weight loss and salt restriction, along with exercise, are usually tried first. Salt restriction is important because high levels of salt in your body can cause you to retain fluids. These fluids can put additional pressure on your blood vessels.

In addition to these measures, medications may be necessary to keep blood pressure in line. Some of these medications, particularly the *thiazide diuretics* and the *beta blockers*, can upset diabetes control. Close medical super-

hiking

vision is crucial if these drugs must be used. In some cases, alternative medicines may be helpful.

If you are taking pills to control your blood pressure, be sure you follow your doctor's and pharmacist's instructions and be sure to take *all* your pills every day.

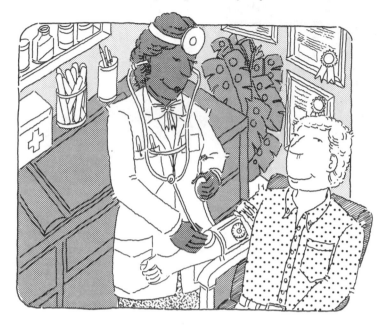

hiking
(HIK-ing)

Take a hike! We don't mean for you to "get lost." Rather, we are suggesting that you get out of the city and enjoy the millions of acres of national parks and forests. Hiking can be a lot of fun, help you reduce stress, and be a great way to get some good aerobic exercise (see Exercise).

Before you hit the trail, get yourself a good pair of sturdy boots or shoes. The type of terrain you will be covering will determine what type of footwear you will need. If you're just going to cover a soft, smooth or paved trail, some good walking or running shoes with good arch supports might do the trick. But if you are going over rough, rocky terrain, you will need some sturdy, waterproof boots. When you have diabetes, you cannot be too careful about care for your feet (see Foot Care). So, buying footwear designed to protect your feet is a wise investment. Also, be sure to break in a new pair of boots or shoes before attempting a long hike.

Like any exercise, you should be careful not to overdo it. If you are thinking of taking a 10-mile hike, don't attempt it until you're ready. Start out by taking short hikes and then work up to longer ones. If you are not used to exercise, you should visit your doctor before you do anything. You may need to take extra precautions or have a health condition that will prevent you from participating in certain activities.

If you take insulin, hike smart. Never hike alone. Let your trailmates know you have diabetes. Teach them how to recognize and treat an insulin reaction. *Always* carry something to treat a reaction, such as some Lifesavers, or a commercially-prepared glucose gel. Hiking burns a lot of calories (about 100 calories per mile on level ground) so you will need to take that into consideration if you take insulin. Be prepared to test your blood-glucose level so you can make food and insulin adjustments along the way.

Make sure your diabetes supplies are packed with you and not with a friend. That way, if you somehow get separated, you will have what you need. If you are venturing out in extreme temperatures, be sure your insulin is protected against the weather. You can pack insulin in some sort of insulated pack to protect it from drastic temperature changes.

The more you prepare for a hike, the better off you will be. You will be free from worry and able to enjoy the serene, peaceful feeling you can get from being close to nature.

history of diabetes
(HIS-tah-ree UV DI-a-BEET-eez)

In India in 3,000 B.C., the physician Susruta described a disease "brought on by gluttonous overindulgence in rice, flour, and sugar," in which urine is "like an elephant's in quantity." A Greek, Aretaeus, in the first century A.D., gave us the word "diabetes." It is from the Greek word for "siphon." After watching some of his patients who had the disease, he noticed that they were very thirsty. Aretaeus thought that their bodies acted like siphons, sucking in water at one end and emptying it at the other.

Ancient physicians knew some of the symptoms of diabetes, but they had no effective way to treat it. Aretaeus recommended dates, raw quinces (a type of fruit), and gruel. As late as 1690, "gelly of viper's flesh," broken red coral, sweet almonds, and "flowers of blind nettles" were prescribed.

Understanding of diabetes progressed faster with the age of scientific experimentation. Thomas Willis, in the 17th century, called doctors' attention to the sweetness of the urine in people with diabetes. In 1776, Dr. Dobson of Liverpool identified the sweetness as sugar. In 1796, Dr. John Rollo, using a urine glucose test devised by Dobson, created the first effective treatment for diabetes. It consisted of a diet high in what he called "animal food"—fat and meat—and low in "vegetable matter"—grains and breads. This diet helped many people with diabetes live longer, and with modifications, was the only treatment for diabetes until the 1920s.

Before proper treatment for type I (insulin-dependent) diabetes was possible, a better understanding of the disease was needed. For many years, no one was sure what part of the body was ill. The stomach, as John Rollo had thought? The kidneys, because of the increased urination? Perhaps the liver? It was not until 1889 that the matter was settled.

That year, two German physiologists, Oskar Minkowski and Joseph von Mering, were investigating the digestion of fat. They knew that the pancreas played a role, so they experimented by removing the pancreases of two dogs. To their surprise, the dogs got diabetes. An article published 23 years before this discovery provided the answer. In that article, Paul Langerhans described some "heaps of cells" in the pancreas

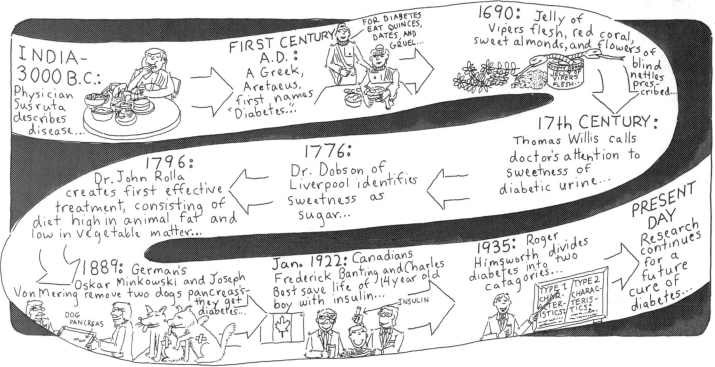

INDIA-3000 B.C.: Physician Susruta describes disease...

FIRST CENTURY A.D.: A Greek, Aretaeus, first names "Diabetes..."

FOR DIABETES EAT QUINCES, DATES, AND GRUEL...

1690: Jelly of Vipers flesh, red coral, sweet almonds, and flowers of blind nettles prescribed...

YUMMY ARAB JELLY OF VIPERS FLESH

17th CENTURY: Thomas Willis calls doctor's attention to sweetness of diabetic urine...

1776: Dr. Dobson of Liverpool identifies sweetness as sugar...

1796: Dr. John Rolla creates first effective treatment, consisting of diet high in animal fat and low in vegetable matter...

1889: German's Oskar Minkowski and Joseph Von Mering remove two dogs pancreas's—they get diabetes...

DOG PANCREAS

Jan. 1922: Canadians Frederick Banting and Charles Best save life of 14 year old boy with insulin...

INSULIN

1935: Roger Himsworth divides diabetes into two catagories...

TYPE 1 CHARACTERISTICS: TYPE 2 CHARACTERISTICS:

PRESENT DAY Research continues for a future cure of diabetes...

for which he could see no function. (Later, these were called the "islets of Langerhans.") Scientists all over the world began searching for the "antidiabetic substance" they thought must be secreted by these cells.

Finally, Canadians Frederick Banting and Charles Best achieved success. They extracted (removed) a substance from the pancreas—insulin—that, when injected into diabetic dogs, lowered the dogs' blood sugar and prevented their death. In January, 1922, Banting and Best tried their extract on Leonard Thompson, a 14-year-old boy dying of diabetes, and saved his life. The insulin era had begun, and for thousands, type I diabetes was no longer as serious a disease.

The history of diabetes since 1921 has not yet been capped off by a discovery as dramatic as that of insulin. However, we do have a greater understanding of diabetes and better treatment than before.

One noteworthy discovery was the realization that diabetes is not a *single* disease. In 1935 Roger Himsworth divided diabetes into two categories: "insulin sensitive" (today called type I) and "insulin insensitive" (the modern type II).

Today, scientists are searching for ways of preventing the complications of diabetes: blindness, kidney failure, gangrene, and heart attacks. And into better insulin delivery: insulin pumps, an artificial pancreas, or pancreas transplants.

One day, the history of diabetes will end with the tale of how diabetes and its complications were cured for good.

holidays

(HALL-a-DAZE)

Thanksgiving, Christmas, Channukah, Easter, Passover—these holidays, once celebrated solely for their spiritual meaning, have become national eating festivals. And

it doesn't stop with just these holidays. The big three-day weekends in the warm weather—Memorial Day, the Fourth of July, and Labor Day—have become picnic marathons of

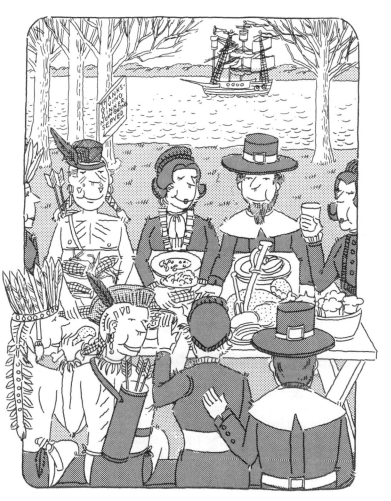

home health care

barbecues, potato salad, and ice cream.

So what is the person with diabetes to do? The first step is to remember that diabetes never takes a holiday. Holiday food feasts always result in higher blood-glucose levels which could lead to increased health risks. Since neither your diabetes nor America's mania for meat, fat, and sugar are likely to disappear overnight, you need to learn how to cope—even during the holidays.

Start before the celebration begins. Eat *before* you go to the party. That way you won't arrive starving and want to grab the first morsel that is put under your nose.

Be careful of proportions when dinner is served. Better yet, help to serve it. Your hostess will appreciate the extra hand, and you will be on your feet burning calories instead of on your behind gulping them. You may even offer to make one of the dishes—something you can eat without guilt and share with friends.

What about dessert? If you can't resist the goodies, don't take more than one helping—and take a small one at that. Better yet, scope out some fruit or nuts or bring some yourself.

Finally, if you know you have overeaten, don't sit there and feel guilty after dinner. Get some exercise right away. Organize a caroling walk, a shell-hunting expedition, or a game of charades with lots of physical activity—depending on the locale and the weather.

Of course, you could save yourself a lot of trouble and have the party at your place. Did we say "*save* yourself a lot of trouble?" Maybe what we meant to say was: Happy Holidays!

home health care
(HOME HELTH KARE)

Have you ever spent some time in the hospital as a patient and wished you could just sit out your illness at home? You're not alone. There are home health agencies across the United States that are providing care in the homes of people who feel the way you do.

Home health care may be the best treatment for you. Studies have shown that people recuperate faster when they are treated at home. And many times it is a lot cheaper than staying in a hospital. Home care is ideal for many people who no longer need the constant care of a hospital but still need minimal care. Home care may even provide an alternative to nursing homes for some people. Of course, there are illnesses that can't be treated anywhere except the hospital. But medical technology has opened up a wide range of health care that can be done in the home.

The actual services you can receive from a home health agency may vary. Services might include any or all of the following: physical, respiratory, occupational, or speech therapy; chemotherapy; nutritional guidance; and personal care like bathing and dressing, even grocery shopping. Agencies may provide blood testing or send in a professional to administer drugs and other treatments. Among the profes-

sionals who may be called on are: a physician, a licensed practical nurse (L.P.N.), a registered nurse (R.N.), a registered dietitian (R.D.), a social worker, a home health aide, a therapist, or a volunteer.

How do you find a home health agency that is best for you? You should first check with your doctor to see if you can be treated at home. Your doctor can also suggest what type of health care would be best for you. He or she might also be able to steer you toward a good agency. Other sources may be your church or synagogue. You might try the United Way or a social service agency for help. Also, don't forget your local American Diabetes Association chapter or affiliate.

Health-care agencies have to be licensed by the state or local governments. The local Health and/or Human Services Department in your state government office might be able to give you some leads also. Some states have home health care associations that provide information on how to find an agency. Check the Yellow Pages of your telephone book under headings such as Health Services, Nursing Services, Visiting Nurse Associations, or Home Health Aides.

Now there is the question of money—how are you going to afford home care? Staying out of the hospital usually saves your insurance company money, so many companies have extended their policies to cover home care. Check with *your* insurance company to see if it covers home care and how much it will pay for. Some may only pay for certain services or only a small portion of home care.

You might also check with the agency to see what financial arrangements you can make with them. They may have a sliding scale of charges so you pay according to your income.

Once you've got that settled, grab your favorite book, fluff up your pillow, and enjoy the quiet of your own home. Oh, and get well soon!

honeymoon phase
(HUN-ee-MOON FAZE)

Insulin-dependent (type I) diabetes plays a nasty trick on about 90 percent of those who develop it. Two to four months after a person starts to take insulin, the person's own islet cells may *temporarily* regain the ability to produce insulin, and the need to inject insulin may go way down. Some people may even be able to stop injecting insulin for a time.

This is the honeymoon phase—also know as *remission*—and it can last anywhere from a month to a year. But like most honeymoons, it does come to an end.

The honeymoon phase, if not recognized for what it is, can do great harm by raising false hopes and by lowering a person's guard against the return of high blood sugar.

If you are the parent of a child going through the honeymoon phase, make it clear that sometimes a person's need for insulin increases and sometimes it decreases. At best, the honeymoon is a vacation from diabetes; a child must know, however, that it lasts only a short time.

hospitals

(HAWS-pi-talz)

Most hospitals do a fine job of handling diabetes—even when you are admitted for reasons other than diabetes control. However, once in a while people do run up against trouble. For example, someone feels an insulin reaction coming on and buzzes the nurse for food, only to be told to wait. . .and wait.

While you may experience problems, chances are good that all will go well if you have to check in a hospital in the future. But the safe health-care consumer is the *careful* health-care consumer. Be prepared for the worst. Some simple precautions can help you ensure that your care will be as good as possible:

■ Before anything happens to you, agree with your doctor on a plan for handling emergencies. Ask what you should do if your doctor is out of town or if you are.

■ Avoid unnecessary surgery. Seek a second opinion when surgery is recommended.

■ Know as much as you can about diabetes. Be sure that a doctor who has a special interest in diabetes is involved in your care during your hospital stay.

■ Ask your physician for a rundown of the events to come. Important questions to ask are, "Will insulin or oral agents be discontinued before surgery?" "How long before?" "When will I start taking the drug again?" If things don't seem to be going according to plan, find out why. It may be an oversight, one that could cost you your comfort and health. If you are too weak to watch over your care, you may want to have a companion do it for you.

■ If you use insulin, work out a plan for handling snacks and insulin reactions and have your doctor put that plan in the written orders. Will you keep food with you or rely on a nurse to bring it to you? Some doctors do not like patients to keep food with them, but others acknowledge that nurses cannot always respond quickly to calls for food from patients with diabetes. If you are used to doing your own blood tests and injections, have orders written that say you can do the same in the hospital.

■ Not satisfied with your care? Depending on the problem, you can call your physician, the hospital dietitian, the nurse in charge of the floor, the social service department, or a patient advocate (ombudsman), if the hospital has one.

If your child is hospitalized:

■ Monitor your child's care as if you were the one in the hospital bed.

■ Arrange to stay in the room overnight if you and your child will feel more secure that way.

hygiene

(HIGH-jean)

Hygiene is the science that deals with the preservation of good health—sounds a lot like good diabetes control, doesn't it? Actually, good personal hygiene should be practiced right along with your diabetes regimen.

A large part of good hygiene involves keeping your body clean. Keeping clean helps get rid of germs that can cause infections. Getting dirt and germs on your hands and other parts of your skin is part of everyday living. Germs grow and multiply on moist, dirty skin. Because many diseases can start with germs on your skin, it's important to keep clean.

Here are a number of hygiene hints:

■ Bathe or shower several times a week. Bathing removes dirt and sweat. Use soap—dirt and sweat cling to the soap, washing off more easily. And don't forget to wash behind your ears! Hair gets dirty, too, so shampoo at least once a week to help keep your scalp and hair clean and healthy. Wash your face at least once a day, too.

■ Dry yourself thoroughly after bathing. People with diabetes are more susceptible to skin problems, especially yeast and fungal infections—conditions which thrive in warm, moist environments. Pay particular attention to body crevices, such as the area between fingers and toes, under arms, the groin, and under the breasts. These are ideal places for fungal growths and yeast infections.

■ Moisturize. Creams or creamy lotions will help keep your skin smooth and supple. Moisturizing helps add and hold moisture in the top layer of the skin. The best time to apply lotion is after you have bathed and lightly toweled off, when your skin is still damp. This way, the lotion "locks in" water, helping to keep skin moist.

■ Wash your hands frequently. Bathing is important for good hygiene, but having clean hands is even more important. Wash your hands, using soap and warm water, before each meal. Most important, wash your hands very well after each time you use the toilet. During the day, many germs will collect on your hands. If you don't wash them off, you'll swallow some with your food. And sooner or later, you'll swallow some germs that can make you sick. After you have washed your hands, be sure to dry them thoroughly on a clean towel.

■ Keep your nails clean. Dirt can collect under fingernails, and anywhere there's dirt, there's bound to be germs. Keep your fingernails cut short. Don't bite them off, though—use nail clippers or scissors. If you keep your nails cut short, it will be that much harder for dirt—and germs—to get under them. Cut your toenails squarely across. Don't go closer to the flesh than the end of the toe, or you risk piercing the skin. (The toenail should be slightly longer than the toe.)

■ Wear clean clothes. The way you dress can be important to health. If you take a bath and then put on dirty clothes, you're putting on the same dirt and germs you just washed off. It's especially important to put on clean underwear and socks after a bath or shower, and to change them each day if you can.

■ Cover your mouth when you sneeze or cough. When you sneeze, many tiny droplets of moisture shoot out into the air. If you have a cold, there are thousands of germs on each droplet. If other people inhale these droplets, they are likely to catch your cold. To prevent this from happening, you should cover your nose with a clean tissue before you sneeze. The tissue will trap the droplets, and hopefully prevent anyone else from catching your cold. Germs can also

hyperglycemia

"escape" when you cough, so you should cover your mouth with your hand when you cough.

Dental hygiene is also important to good health. People with diabetes are especially susceptible to tooth and gum disease, and need to pay extra attention to dental care. Plaque—a sticky, colorless substance—builds up on your teeth due to the foods you eat. Plaque is the perfect resting place for bacteria. Bacteria stick to the plaque and cause food particles to ferment, producing acid. This acid can eat through the hard enamel that protects the outside of the tooth. If the acid eats far enough into the tooth, a cavity is formed. If enough plaque builds up, it forms a hard substance called tartar. Tartar can only be removed by your dentist—it must be scraped off. Excess tartar can cause gum disease (periodontal disease) and lead to loss of teeth. Follow these rules for good dental care:

■ Brush your teeth thoroughly at least twice a day. Use toothpaste. It is even better if you brush several times a day, especially after meals and snacks. Brush your tongue, too—food particles can also hide there.

■ Floss in between teeth. Flossing removes food particles from areas that your brush cannot reach. It is just as important as brushing for keeping your teeth and gums healthy.

■ See your dentist regularly. Professional cleaning of the teeth is important because your dentist can do a more thorough job of cleaning your teeth than you. Also, your dentist can check the condition of your teeth and gums for signs of decay or disease.

Because hygiene involves preserving health, there are several other things you can do to help keep yourself healthy. Follow your diabetes regimen—your meal plan, exercise, and medication are your most important tools for staying healthy. Don't smoke, and get a good night's rest (sleep is important for good health, too). Practicing good hygiene isn't difficult nor is it expensive—it's just a wise investment toward good health.

hyperglycemia
(HI-per-gli-see-me-ah)

High blood sugar (hyperglycemia) happens when the body has too little, or not enough, insulin, or when too much food is eaten. Insulin moves sugar from the blood into the body cells. Without insulin, sugar collects in your blood. In general, a blood level reading of 180 mg/dl is considered hyperglycemic and is undesirable for diabetes control.

You can have high blood sugar for a number of reasons. You may not have given yourself a sufficient dosage of insulin. Or you might have eaten more than you planned, or exercised less than planned. Maybe you're going through some physical stress (such as illness, trauma, or infection) or emotional difficulties (such as family conflicts or on-going school or dating problems). All these things can contribute to hyperglycemia.

You may recognize the symptoms of hyperglycemia—they are the same classic symptoms of diabetes: elevated blood-sugar levels, high levels of sugar in the urine, increased urina-tion, and increased thirst.

How do you prevent hyperglycemia? We bet you know the answer. Yep, proper diabetes control. Self-monitoring of blood glucose is the best prevention. Frequent testing allows you to spot and treat high blood sugar before any symptoms appear. We don't want to seem like a nag, but don't forget to also follow your meal plan and to exercise.

Exercise sometimes is helpful in lowering high blood sugar sufficiently. However, if your blood-glucose level is above 250 mg/dl, don't exercise. When your blood-glucose level is above 250 mg/dl, exercise may only help to raise it even higher. Also, if you are planning on exercising, be sure to check for ketones first (if blood glucose is more than 240 mg/dl). If ketones are present, *don't exercise*.

Limiting the amount of food you eat might also help avoid hyperglycemia. If following your meal plan and exercising don't work, adjusting your insulin dosage might.

Be sure to talk with your doctor. He or she should be able to help you pinpoint the problem and make adjustments in your diabetes care plan.

The best thing you can remember is not to get "hyper." Instead, get smart and keep your diabetes in control.

hyperosmolar nonketotic coma
(hi-per-oz-MOE-lar non-key-TOT-ick KO-ma)

If you peeked ahead and read about ketoacidosis, you learned about one type of diabetic coma. Hyperosmolar is another type of diabetic coma. Like ketoacidosis, hyperosmolar nonketotic coma comes on gradually. Hyperosmolar coma can kill you if not treated promptly. Most often, that treatment must be done in a hospital.

Unlike ketoacidosis, hyperosmolar coma occurs almost exclusively among elderly people with *non*-insulin dependent diabetes. It is seldom accompanied by ketones in the urine (which is why it is also known as *nonketotic* coma).

Because hyperosmolar coma is a life-threatening condition, elderly people with diabetes and their family members should be alert to its symptoms. Chief among them is dehydration—generally marked by extreme thirst and frequent urination. When blood sugar rises to extremely high levels, it causes water to be drawn away from cells and tissues. The extra water, along with excess glucose, is released through the urine. (The word "hyperosmolar" refers to the chemical changes that draw water from body tissues to the blood.)

Other symptoms include:
■ weakness
■ fatigue
■ high amounts of glucose in urine and blood
■ dry mouth
■ shallow breathing
■ flushed, dry skin
■ confusion
■ drowsiness

Hyperosmolar coma most often appears after an event that raises blood-sugar levels, such as an accident, an acute illness or infection, a stroke, or physical or emotional stress. Other possible triggers include taking large doses of drugs that raise blood sugar (such as steroids, diuretics, and some tranquilizers), and poor kidney function.

Treatment for hyperosmolar coma must always be given in a hospital. There, insulin will be administered, lost fluids will be replaced, and blood sugar carefully monitored. *Do not try to treat it yourself.* However, if a person suffering from hyperosmolar coma is conscious and asks for water, it is safe to give as much as he or she wants before help arrives. The water will help to counter the severe dehydration.

hypoglycemia
(hi-po-gli-SEE-me-ah)

You start the day feeling good. You decide to go outside to work in the yard. While you are working, you begin to tremble; your hands begin to perspire; you get dizzy; your pulse rises—you may be experiencing hypoglycemia (also known as an insulin reaction).

Hypoglycemia is low blood sugar (*hypo*— low, *glyc*—sugar, and *emia*—blood). This drop in blood sugar could bring on the following symptoms:
- behavior changes
- numbness in the arms and hands
- inattention or confusion
- tingling sensations around the mouth
- shakiness or dizziness
- sweating
- faintness
- increased pulse rate
- irritability
- clumsy or jerky movements
- pale skin color
- headache
- moodiness
- hunger

Common causes of insulin reactions include:
- Doing strenuous exercise without eating a snack beforehand (half a sandwich is good). Exercise lowers your blood sugar by causing the sugar to move from the blood into the muscles.
- Taking too much insulin.
- Eating too little food, such as when you delay or skip a meal.
- Eating too much and then compensating with a too-high dose of insulin.
- Drinking alcohol on an empty stomach.

While you'll want to avoid the above problems, you also have to maintain a balance of your meal plan, exercise, and insulin. Recognize that it is difficult, if not impossible, to always do the same amount of activity and eat the same amount of food at the same exact time every day. Even if you did, your body might still respond differently at different

times and you could have an insulin reaction anyway. In fact, anyone who takes insulin is bound to have reactions now and then. However, if you have frequent reactions, see your doctor. You may need a change in your treatment plan.

When you first feel the symptoms of a reaction, you should test to see what your blood-glucose level is. If it is low, *treat* it with some form of quick-acting sugar. Things you could take to treat a reaction are: sugar cubes, honey, orange juice, candy, or a nondiet soft drink. Glucose tablets, liquids, and gels are also made specifically for treating reactions. You need not overdo the sugar. Usually about 10 grams of simple carbohydrate (see Carbohydrates) is enough. This equals about four ounces of orange juice, four Life Savers, or half a candy bar. Many people who have had diabetes for many years say that eventually each person finds the one food that really treats his or her reactions. For some people, it's milk; for others, it's orange slices.

After 10 or 15 minutes, test your blood-glucose level again. If your blood glucose is still low and your symptoms don't go away, repeat the treatment. Once you feel better, eat some protein such as cheese, a glass of milk, or a meat sandwich. This will help to keep your blood-glucose level up.

Sometimes insulin users have such bad reactions that they pass out. You need to be prepared for such a reaction. To protect yourself in case you become unconscious, get a glucagon kit. Glucagon is a hormone that raises blood sugar. Glucagon is only available by prescription, so ask your doctor to prescribe it for you. It would be a good idea to keep glucagon at home and at work. Also, you need to be sure a family member or roommate, and a co-worker know how to inject glucagon should you need it.

(Note: People cannot always tell whether you have passed out because of high or low blood sugar. Let them know that if they have any doubts about your condition they should give you glucagon (**never insulin**) and call your doctor or the nearest hospital. If sugar is already high, a little more probably won't make much difference. But when glucose is very low, it must be raised quickly to avoid brain damage or even death. Let friends and co-workers know that treating a non-reaction is safer than failing to treat a real one. The motto should be: When in doubt, treat with sugar.)

IDs
(i-DENT-a-fi-kay-shuns)

Don't leave home without them. When you have diabetes, an identification card can be more important than your credit cards. You should wear and carry some form of identification. (This is because police in some places are prohibited from searching an unconscious person's pocket or wallet.)

A bracelet or necklace that says, "I have diabetes" will alert police, paramedics, or hospital personnel in case of an emergency. Remember that the symptoms of an insulin reaction may be mistaken for drunkenness. Proper identification will set people straight and help ensure that you receive the treatment you need. Bracelets and necklaces are

immunosuppression

available through Medic Alert of Turlock, California, and most pharmacies.

You should also carry a card in your wallet with your name, address, and phone number, and those of your physician. An emergency is no time to trust important phone numbers to memory. Your card should also show the type of insulin or oral drug you take, the dosage, and the time of day you take it. Identification cards are available from your local American Diabetes Association affiliate or chapter.

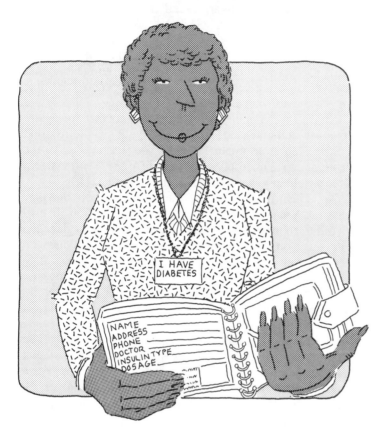

immunosuppression

(IM-myoo-no-sah-PRESH-un)

The immune system is the body's defense against outside invaders such as viruses and bacteria, which can cause infections. To protect the body, the immune system has a host of "soldiers" armed with T-cells and antibodies to destroy these invaders. In type I diabetes, these soldiers somehow get an incorrect message to destroy the beta cells of the pancreas. (The beta cells are the insulin producers.) This misguided attack is called an *autoimmune reaction* because the body has turned on itself (*auto* means self).

What triggers these immune system soldiers to attack the beta cells is unknown. But researchers have suggested that stopping the soldiers from completing the attack may stop the onset of diabetes. And that's what immunosuppression is all about: preventing the immune system soldiers from completing their destruction of the beta cells. This is done by sup-

pressing (holding back) the immune system (thus, the term *immunosuppression*).

Immunosuppression is presently used strictly in research settings and only on people whose diabetes is newly diagnosed. That's because in general, these people still have *some* functioning beta cells. These individuals are given powerful drugs that prevent the immune system from working. The idea is to stop the immune system at this point so that the remaining beta cells are not destroyed. This could then reduce or eliminate the need for insulin. But this therapy is still experimental and there are many hurdles to overcome before it is commonly used.

For example, holding back the immune system weakens the system and leaves individuals open to an increased risk of infection. And the drugs (cyclosporin is one) used to suppress the immune system have some harmful side effects, ranging from nausea and abnormalities of white blood cell production, to kidney damage and an increased risk of cancer.

Research is ongoing to find a better way of stopping the immune system's soldiers from attacking the beta cells without leaving people open to infection and harmful side effects.

impaired glucose tolerance

(im-PAIRED GLOO-kose TALL-er-ans)

Latent, borderline, or chemical diabetes are terms that once were used for a condition that is now called *impaired glucose tolerance*. This condition is no longer considered a form of diabetes.

If you are given this diagnosis, it means that your blood sugar falls between "normal" and "diabetic" levels. A person with impaired glucose tolerance does, however, have an increased risk of developing diabetes.

One way impaired glucose tolerance is discovered is through a test called a glucose tolerance test (see Blood Tests). If you were having this test performed, you would be asked to fast (not eat) for eight to 12 hours. You would then have a sample of your blood taken (a fasting sample). Then you would be asked to drink a glucose solution. Your blood sugar would then be tested at regular intervals to see how your body handles sugar.

After all the samples are drawn, your doctor would chart the results on a graph. If the curve shows a rise in your glucose level and then returns to normal within about three hours, you do not have diabetes. If the curve shows an abnormally high rise in your glucose level and then gradually returns to normal, you may have impaired glucose tolerance. Impaired glucose tolerance is when your blood-sugar curve falls in between the normal and diabetic range.

Once you are diagnosed, your doctor will want to help you correct impaired glucose tolerance so it won't develop into diabetes. Your doctor will probably start you out on an appropriate exercise and meal plan. He or she may also work to help you lose weight, if necessary. After a period of time, your doctor will want to test you again to see if you have made any progress or if you have developed diabetes.

implantable pumps
(im-PLANT-able PUMPS)

Ever since the first insulin injection, researchers have been experimenting with different ways to get insulin from the bottle to the bloodstream. One of the latest—and still highly experimental—advances in insulin delivery is the implantable pump. This device is so small and sophisticated that it is actually worn *under* the skin.

Several different kinds of implantable insulin pumps have now been tested on people, but the "perfect" pump hasn't been invented yet. Scientists are working to make the pumps more closely resemble the function of a pancreas. The ideal pump will include a reservoir to hold the insulin and a pump to deliver the insulin. Once perfected, it will also have a sensor to monitor blood-glucose levels. This monitoring is necessary to make sure that the right amounts of insulin are released to meet the body's needs.

Scientists have been testing an implantable device that is about the size of a hockey puck (about 3 inches in diameter and less than 1 inch thick). The device is surgically implanted in the abdomen (stomach area). Because it has a sizable insulin reservoir, refills are only necessary four to five times a year. This device does not have to be programmed manually. A doctor can adjust insulin flow with by using a radio transmitter. However, the pump does not have a glucose sensor. Thus, the person using it will still have to monitor blood-glucose levels.

Until there is a cure for diabetes, implantable pumps may be an option for some people in helping them control their diabetes. If you have diabetes, you may want to keep up-to-date on the latest technology. Your American Diabetes Association affiliate and chapter, and *Diabetes Forecast* are good sources to turn to for new diabetes information.

impotence
(IM-po-tens)

Because you have diabetes does not mean you can't have an active sex life. Diabetes does not make sex any less pleasurable. However, diabetes may diminish a man's ability to achieve an erection. Over one-third of all men who have diabetes are impotent. But, diabetes is not the cause of impotence in all impotent men with diabetes—impotence can be caused by a host of factors, not the least of which is frame of mind. Simply stated, impotence is the inability to have or sustain an erection.

One cause of impotence in men with diabetes is neuropathy (nerve damage). When a man is aroused, the pelvic nerves activate the arteries in the penis and they expand. This allows

more blood to flow in and make the penis erect. However, when there is damage to the pelvic nerves, they may not work properly, or not at all. If the pelvic nerves are not working properly, a man will have difficulty achieving or sustaining an erection.

Another cause of impotence in men with diabetes is blockage of the penile artery. This artery is medium-sized, much like those arteries that supply blood to the heart. When the penile artery is blocked, less blood is allowed to enter the penis, hampering the ability to sustain an erection. The odds for this happening increase as a man ages, particularly if diabetes is poorly controlled.

Certain medications can also cause impotence. For example, antihypertensive agents—drugs that are used to help control high blood pressure—are also known to cause impotence. (Propranonol and methyldopa are two types of these agents.)

You should discuss any problems you have with a medication with your doctor. You *should not* stop taking any drugs without first talking with your doctor. If medication is making you impotent, it is likely you and your doctor will be able to find a solution.

What can you do to prevent impotence? First, don't worry—fear of becoming impotent can sometimes be the cause. Just knowing that diabetes is associated with impotence may scare some men into becoming impotent. Stress can be a big factor in causing impotence. If your problems are psychological, a reputable counselor should be able to help you. Counseling can help you correct misconceptions, restore openness, and teach sensual alternatives to sexual intercourse.

If you have diabetes, there are precautions you can take to avoid becoming impotent. One, take control of your diabetes. While it is not conclusive, it is likely that good control of your blood-glucose levels will help you avoid becoming impotent. Good control may help you avoid some of the physical ailments mentioned before (neuropathy, blocked blood vessels). Also, if you are in control, you will feel better and if you feel better, your sex life may be better.

You should also avoid drinking excessive amounts of alcohol. Studies have shown drinking large amounts of alcohol can cause impotence. And, don't smoke. Smoking causes blood vessels to constrict (narrow) and this contributes to artery blockages. As we said before, blockage of arteries can cause impotence.

What hope is there for the man who is impotent? One effective method is the penile prosthesis. There are two main types. Both have two hollow cylinders which are surgically placed inside the penis. One type is called semi-rigid. This type of prothesis has a core of silver wire or stainless steel. It can be bent to a flaccid (limp) or erect position. It can be put in under a local anesthetic. It is the cheaper of the two devices.

The other type is called an inflatable prosthesis. It has a pumping device that can be activated whenever a man would like to have an erection. Placement of this prothesis is done under a general anesthesia.

Another method used to help men produce an erection is a vacuum pump. This is how it works: A container is placed over the penis. A pump then draws all the air out of the container, creating a vacuum. This vacuum produces an erec-

infection

tion. Before removing the container, a rubber band must be placed around the base of the penis to maintain the erection. (The rubber band cannot be worn indefinitely. After 20 minutes, the rubber band could damage the penis by bruising it.)

Physicians have found that certain drugs injected into the penis will produce an erection. Two of the most common drugs are papaverine and phentolamine. Although successful, side effects may include bruising and persistent erections that can last several hours. An oral medication, yohimbine, may help to increase penis rigidity; unfortunately, it may worsen high blood pressure. As with all drugs, you should discuss them and their side effects with your doctor.

Impotence is a complication of diabetes. Because it is, you should do all you can to beat the odds of it happening to you. However, even if you are experiencing impotence, you still can have a sex life—a lot of it depends on how inventive you and your partner are.

infection

(in-FEK-shun)

Remember how you felt when that nasty cold was coming on last winter? Your body was being invaded by tiny organisms that were multiplying rapidly, making you feel worse by the hour. To fight this invasion, the body produced antibodies, or had an "immunological" response. Battling infections can place stress on all body systems. For people with diabetes, stress caused by an infection anywhere in the body can disrupt diabetes control.

Infections in people with diabetes commonly occur in the urinary tract (inflammation of the bladder or of the renal pelvis); the lungs (flu and pneumonia); the skin (boils and carbuncles); the legs and feet; and the mouth (tooth and gum problems). While these kinds of infections are not necessarily more frequent among persons with diabetes, when they do occur, they are often more serious and last longer.

Prevention is the watchword. Take good care of your teeth and gums, your skin, and particularly your feet—your feet are farthest from the heart, the source of the blood supply. (See Dental Care, Foot Care, and Skin.) Report *any* infection to your doctor, even if it seems minor to you. Also, test blood frequently during infections for high blood-glucose levels, and urine for ketones. If ketones are present and glucose is high, you may be headed for ketoacidosis (see Ketoacidosis).

injections

(in-JEK-shuns)

Daily injections aren't fun to think about, much less receive. But they are necessary.

While you can't expect pleasure from your injections, there are things you can do to make them easier and less painful.

Equipment and technique make a difference. Here are some tips to make injections easier:

■ First, be sure you're using the right size syringe. Syringes come in three sizes and your doctor will prescribe yours based on your insulin needs. Also, make sure that if you're using U-100 insulin, that's what your syringe is designed for. The wrong size syringe can sometimes account for poor control. This is because if you are using the wrong size syringe, your insulin dose may be incorrect.

■ The most comfortable and convenient are the disposable syringes with lubricated "micro-fine" needles that help ensure smooth penetration. While glass syringes and replaceable needles are slightly cheaper, they require careful cleaning and don't slide through the skin as easily.

■ Injecting cold insulin can cause discomfort. Take your current bottle of insulin out of the refrigerator about 30 minutes before injection. After your injection, return the bottle to the refrigerator, and store all extra bottles in the refrigerator. You should discuss storage of your insulin with your pharmacist periodically.

■ Pinch a fold of skin between your thumb and forefinger and inject into it, rather than just stabbing at flat skin. Or, if you use an arm, roll the "flab" against the back of a chair. If you can pinch more than one inch of flab, you can insert the needle straight in (at 90 degrees to the skin). If you pinch less than one inch, insert the needle at a 45-degree angle.

■ Putting the needle in quickly, using a dart-throwing motion, frequently helps. Hesitation only hurts. After the needle is through the skin, push the plunger down to inject the insulin. Again, a rapid push minimizes discomfort. Fast action is also best for removal.

■ Finally, after the injection, cover the site with cotton and apply slight pressure for five to eight seconds. *Do not rub*, since this may cause the insulin to be absorbed too quickly and might irritate the skin.

insulin

(IN-soo-lin)

Less than a century ago, insulin, as a drug, was first used to treat people with diabetes. And since its discovery as a diabetes treatment in 1921, and its first commercial use two years later, insulin has done a lot of growing up.

From 1921 to 1936, the only form of insulin made for injection was rapid-acting, "Regular" insulin. This insulin was extracted from the pancreases of pigs and cows. It had to be injected before each meal and at bedtime. In 1936, protamine zinc insulin (PZI), the first long-acting insulin, was introduced. PZI, which is no longer used, was slower acting and lasted longer in the body than other insulins that were produced years later.

Neutral Protamine Hagedorn (NPH) insulin, named after the Danish researcher who developed it, was introduced in 1950. NPH acted faster than PZI and remained in the bloodstream longer than Regular insulin. Lente insulin was the next development in modified insulins. Introduced in 1954, Lente worked much like NPH, but contained no prota-

insulin

Product	Manufacturer	Form	Strength
Rapid acting (onset 1/2–2 hours)			
Humulin R (Regular)	Lilly	Human	U-100
Iletin I Regular	Lilly	Beef/Pork	U-100
Iletin II Regular	Lilly	Pork	U-100, U-500
Novolin R (Regular)	Novo Nordisk	Human	U-100
Novolin R Penfill (Regular)	Novo Nordisk	Human	U-100
Purified Pork R (Regular)	Novo Nordisk	Pork	U-100
Regular	Novo Nordisk	Pork	U-100
Velosulin Human (Regular)(Buffered)	Novo Nordisk	Human	U-100
Intermediate acting (onset 2–4 hours)			
Humulin L (Lente)	Lilly	Human	U-100
Humulin N (NPH)	Lilly	Human	U-100
Iletin I Lente	Lilly	Beef/Pork	U-100
Iletin I NPH	Lilly	Beef/Pork	U-100
Iletin II Lente	Lilly	Pork	U-100
Iletin II NPH	Lilly	Pork	U-100
Lente	Novo Nordisk	Beef	U-100
Novolin L (Lente)	Novo Nordisk	Human	U-100
Novolin N (NPH)	Novo Nordisk	Human	U-100
Novolin N PenFill (NPH)	Novo Nordisk	Human	U-100
NPH	Novo Nordisk	Beef	U-100
Purified Pork Lente	Novo Nordisk	Pork	U-100
Purified Pork N (NPH)	Novo Nordisk	Pork	U-100
Long acting (onset 4–6 hours)			
Humulin U (Ultralente)	Lilly	Human	U-100
Ultralente	Novo Nordisk	Beef	U-100
Mixtures			
Humulin 50/50 (50% NPH, 50% Regular)	Lilly	Human	U-100
Humulin 70/30 (70% NPH, 30% Regular)	Lilly	Human	U-100
Novolin 70/30 (70% NPH, 30% Regular)	Novo Nordisk	Human	U-100
Novolin 70/30 Penfill (70% NPH, 30% Regular)	Novo Nordisk	Human	U-100
Novolin 70/30 Prefilled (70% NPH, 30% Regular)	Novo Nordisk	Human	U-100

insulin reaction

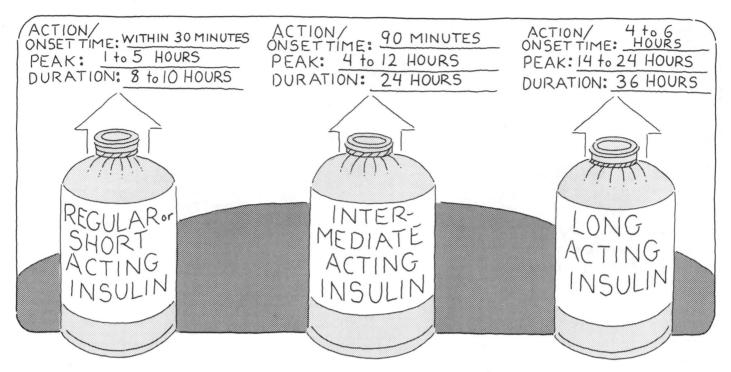

ACTION/ONSET TIME: WITHIN 30 MINUTES	ACTION/ONSET TIME: 90 MINUTES	ACTION/ONSET TIME: 4 to 6 HOURS
PEAK: 1 to 5 HOURS	PEAK: 4 to 12 HOURS	PEAK: 14 to 24 HOURS
DURATION: 8 to 10 HOURS	DURATION: 24 HOURS	DURATION: 36 HOURS
REGULAR or SHORT ACTING INSULIN	INTER-MEDIATE ACTING INSULIN	LONG ACTING INSULIN

mine. Protamine was found to contribute to allergic reactions in some people.

From 1936 to 1972, the insulin being produced was about 85 to 98 percent pure with other products being produced with the insulin. After 1972, purer insulins were developed using gel-filtration chromatography and, later, ion-exchange chromatography as well. These two new manufacturing steps, when used together, result in highly purified insulins that are 99.999 percent pure. Purer insulins seem to cause fewer allergic reactions and they seem to be absorbed into the bloodstream better and work better.

Now "human" insulin is on the market. This insulin is chemically identical to that produced by the human pancreas; however, it is produced in a laboratory. There are two types. One is the semisynthetic. This type is made by converting pork insulin. The other form is synthetic, sometimes called recombinant or rDNA. This form is identical to human insulin and is made through genetic engineering.

Now that we've given you some history, let's talk insulin talk. First, there are some key words that will help you understand action time. Action time is the time it takes the insulin to reach your bloodstream and affect your blood-glucose level. *Onset* is when the insulin begins to affect the blood-glucose level. It can take from 30 minutes to 4 to 6 hours depending on the person and the type of insulin. *Peak* is the time when the insulin is most effective at lowering your blood-glucose level. *Duration* is how long the insulin remains in your bloodstream.

Now for lesson two: The types of insulin. The first kind is Regular or short-acting insulin. It usually reaches the bloodstream quickly (within 30 minutes). This insulin peaks from 1 to 5 hours after injection and will remain in the bloodstream about 8 to 10 hours.

The next type is intermediate-acting (NPH or Lente) insulin. It takes about 90 minutes for this type of insulin to reach the blood. It peaks after 4 to 12 hours and has a duration of up to 24 hours.

Long-acting (Ultralente) insulins take 4 to 6 hours to reach the bloodstream. They are strongest 14 to 24 hours after injection. This type of insulin is often used in combination with Regular insulin in multiple-injection therapy (four or more injections a day).

As we mentioned, insulin is made from different sources: beef, pork, beef-pork combinations, and human insulins. The source of insulin has little to do with how it works to lower blood sugar. But the source can make a difference in how quickly the insulin is absorbed. Recent studies indicate that human insulins are absorbed by the body quicker than beef or pork mixtures.

Also, some insulins—most notably those from beef and the older, less pure beef-pork insulins—can cause an allergic reaction, such as redness or pitting at the injection sites (remember the protamine?). If this happens, you may need to switch insulins. DO NOT switch insulins without talking to your doctor first. With his or her advice, you'll be able to make an informed decision and you'll know what to look for when you switch.

insulin reaction

(IN-soo-lin re-AK-shun)

See Hypoglycemia

insulin resistance

(IN-soo-lin ree-ZIS-tens)

Your pancreas and liver work as a team. When everything is working right, your liver produces enough glucose to give your body the energy it needs to keep going. Your pancreas secretes insulin to move that glucose into cells. Your liver, sensing the rising insulin level, slows its production of glucose. As the glucose production drops, your pancreas slows the amount of insulin it produces.

But for most people with type II diabetes this system breaks down. Most of the time, the liver and pancreas continue to produce glucose and insulin as before. The problem is that the liver as well as the muscles and the fat cells don't respond properly to the insulin. They ignore the insulin, or more technically, they become "resistant" to it. When this happens the liver can't sense the rising insulin level. So, it continues to make more glucose. As your blood-glucose level rises, your pancreas senses the glucose and continues to secrete insulin. Eventually, your liver and pancreas do work things out and stop the production cycle. Still, they are keeping each other in check at levels too high to be good for your body. Your body doesn't handle high levels of glucose in the blood very well for long periods of time. Also, new evidence indicates that the body has a hard time handling large amounts of insulin.

Researchers are not sure what causes insulin resistance, but there are some clues. One big area of study is receptors. Receptors are sensitive areas on a cell's surface. These receptors are the keyholes into which insulin, the key, must fit. But the keyhole is only part of the lock. All of the internal workings of the receptor, or the lock mechanism, must be in full working order. For unknown reasons, obesity—particularly obesity combined with inactivity—causes insulin receptors to stop working or become resistant to insulin action: The lock no longer recognizes the key. Too much insulin in the blood also causes the receptors to shut down. In other words, the keys have entered the keyholes, but are unable to open the door because the lock mechanism is not working properly. This means there are fewer doorways for the insulin and glucose to enter. Because the insulin doesn't have anywhere to go, both insulin and blood-glucose levels rise.

For people with type II diabetes, weight loss and regular exercise seem to help solve the insulin-receptor problem. Therefore, exercise and weight control are *very* real treatments for people with type II diabetes.

insurance
(in-SURE-ens)

Having diabetes does not exclude you from getting insurance, though sometimes it may be difficult. One problem is finding an affordable policy to meet your needs. Group plans for both life and health/major medical are easiest to get into, usually offer the best benefits, and have the most reasonable rates. These are usually offered through your employer.

If you are not eligible for group insurance, you can obtain individual coverage, but it will be more costly. Select several insurance companies, examine the plans they offer and then make a trial application to one of them. Should your applica-

tion be refused, you are still free to apply elsewhere.

When you find a company willing to insure you and a policy that meets your needs, submit a firm application. Be honest—don't try to hide that you have diabetes. Major medical policies should be examined carefully for their rules on reimbursing treatments for pre-existing conditions, and for the size of their deductibles (the amount of the medical bill you pay before the insurance company starts to cover you). Usually, the higher the deductible, the lower the premium (monthly insurance payment).

When selecting life insurance, study the advantages *to you* for term versus whole life. Term insurance is purchased for a set number of years, after which the policy must be renewed. Whole life remains in effect until your death. While whole life insurance may cost more, your coverage cannot be discontinued (unless you fail to pay your premiums). An insuror may refuse to renew a term policy.

Some states have high-risk major medical insurance available to persons with chronic disease who cannot get insurance elsewhere. Check to see if your state has such a plan or has one in the works. Premiums on these policies are comparable to those of other individual policies.

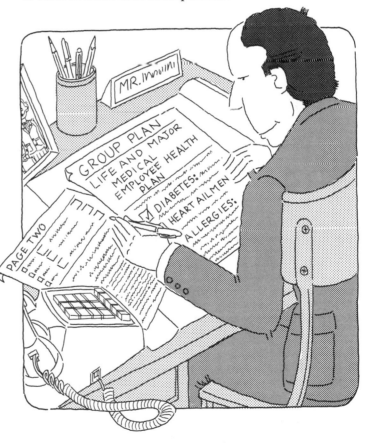

jobs
(JOBS)

Employers are not allowed to fire or refuse employment to a person solely because he or she has diabetes—at least under most conditions. If you are qualified for a job and your diabetes does not prevent you from effectively performing

jogging

your work, there is no reason you should not be hired.

The federal government and some state laws protect a person in many cases against job discrimination. Title V of the federal law called the Rehabilitation Act of 1973 protects the rights of anyone who works for the federal government, for institutions that receive federal funds, or for employers with

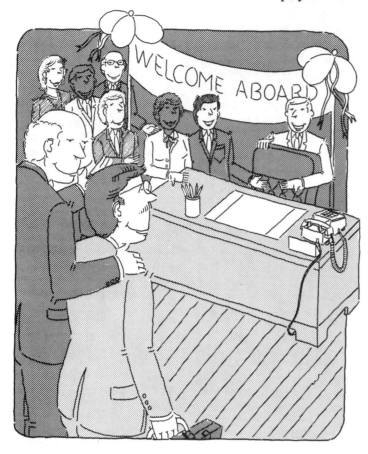

federal contracts of more than $2,500. In addition, most states have laws that protect people in that state regardless of the company they work for. People with diabetes may not consider themselves "handicapped," but they are protected by the laws guarding the rights of the handicapped.

The American Diabetes Association's position on employment is: Diabetes as such should not be a cause for discriminating against any person in employment. People with diabetes should be individually considered for employment weighing such factors as the requirements or hazards of the specific job, and the individual's medical condition and treatment regimen (diet, oral hypoglycemic agents, and insulin). Any person with diabetes, whether insulin-dependent or non-insulin-dependent, should be eligible for any employment for which he or she is otherwise qualified.

In other words, you should not shy away from any job you think is right for you. However, if you know that your health is likely to put you or others in jeopardy in a particular job, common sense dictates that you steer clear of that position. Further, some fields may be barred to you by law. For instance, people with diabetes are not allowed to enter the armed forces.

If you feel you have been discriminated against, first discuss the problem informally with the employer. If that fails, you can file a formal grievance (the personnel office will give you details). You can also have a lawyer explain your concerns to the employer. In addition, check into the state laws that protect you.

If you work for the government, your first step is to contact the Equal Employment Opportunity (EEO) counselor at the workplace. This person should be able to explain the options you have.

If you work for a federal contractor, contact the local or regional office of the Office of Federal Contract Compliance Programs (OFCCP). Check the phone book under the "U.S. Department of Labor."

If you work for an institution receiving federal funds, contact the federal agencies that provide the money.

Generally, employers cannot legally ask you if you have diabetes before hiring you. But an employer may ask you how your health is or if there are any limitations the company should be aware of. You may want to tell your employer at the start to avoid any sticky situations. Another tactic would be to wait until you employer can see how well you work and that your diabetes does not get in the way of your job performance. You should eventually tell your employer you have diabetes. To avoid any problems in case you have an insulin reaction, it is always a good idea to let a co-worker know you have diabetes, and how to help you if you do have a reaction.

Now, put on your best clothes, stand up straight, and charge ahead to the job hunt.

jogging
(JAWG-ing)

See Running

ketoacidosis
(key-toe-ass-i-DOE-sis)

One of the most serious outcomes of poorly controlled diabetes is ketoacidosis, often called *diabetic coma*. The condition, which occurs almost exclusively in people with type I diabetes, is marked by high blood-sugar levels along with high levels of sugar and ketones in the urine.

Although it is accompanied by high blood sugar, ketoacidosis is not *caused* by high blood sugar. It is caused by a lack of insulin. Without insulin, sugar has no way to enter and fuel the body's cells. The fuel is what gives your body the energy to perform the daily tasks of life. When insulin—and therefore sugar—is not available, the body breaks down fats to get that fuel. In the process of breaking down fats, acid substances called *ketone bodies* are released. As the acid levels rise, the body tries to get rid of the ketone bodies through the urine. If acid continues to build up in the blood, it can kill you.

Unlike insulin reactions, ketoacidosis usually develops gradually—often over a period of hours. (When vomiting occurs, however, ketones can develop in about four hours.) Causes of ketoacidosis may include neglected diabetes management, an unexpected stress—such as illness—that increases the need for insulin, and undiagnosed diabetes. Immediate treatment by a doctor is essential. The warning signs may include a dry mouth, thirst (but not hunger), nausea, and excessive urination. The skin is dry and flushed, breathing labored, and the breath has a fruity odor (caused by ketones). Sometimes there is vomiting, abdominal pain, and—if advanced—unconsciousness.

As you can see, ketoacidosis is a condition to be taken seriously and treated as soon as it is detected. By recognizing the symptoms and testing your urine regularly (see Urine Tests), you can help prevent ketoacidosis from happening to you.

ketones

(KEY-tones)

See Ketoacidosis

kidneys

(KID-neez)

Normal kidneys are only about the size of a baking potato, but they have a big role to play in the body—they keep toxic waste products in our blood at low levels.

A brief overview of how your kidneys work should give you a better appreciation for these remarkable organs. Your body breaks down protein as you eat. As your body digests your food, waste products gradually build up in your blood. While this is happening, blood containing these waste products enters your kidneys. There, millions of tiny blood vessels act as filters to remove wastes, chemicals, and excess water from the blood. These filters then pass the waste products into the urine. Important parts of your blood, such as red blood cells, are too big to pass through these tiny filters, and so they remain in the blood. Very little blood protein is allowed to pass into the urine by a kidney that is functioning normally.

When these filters become damaged, however, they become leaky and let protein spill into the blood. (Think of a screen with a hole punched through it.) Eventually, these filters wear away and no longer exist. When this happens, more stress is put on the remaining filters and they eventually become damaged. This causes the kidney to become less and less efficient. When the entire filtration system breaks down, your kidneys fail to function.

Kidney failure is a complication of diabetes and can be life-threatening. Your doctor should check the functioning of your kidneys periodically. Through blood and urine tests, your doctor can tell if your kidneys are functioning properly.

If you are diagnosed with kidney failure (nephropathy), you and your doctor will need to decide on a method of therapy. Two methods of therapy are available: dialysis

and transplantation.

Dialysis is a process where the blood is cleansed by a kidney substitute. This is the more common form of treatment for kidney failure. There are two types of dialysis. *Hemodialysis* is the first method. In this process, a person's blood (drawn from a vein in the person's arm) is circulated through a machine. The machine removes waste products and then returns the blood back to the body. This process may be done in a hospital setting and takes three to five hours. It must be done three days a week. *Peritoneal dialysis* is the other method. This process does not require the blood to go through a machine. Rather, the blood is passed through the person's abdominal cavity (called the peritoneum). A small catheter is permanently placed through a tiny hole in the abdomen. A special fluid is passed in and out of the abdominal cavity through the catheter. The waste products from the blood are drawn from the fluid and are later discarded.

Transplantation of a healthy kidney to replace a damaged one is becoming more and more popular. Transplantation frees a person from dialysis and improves the quality of life.

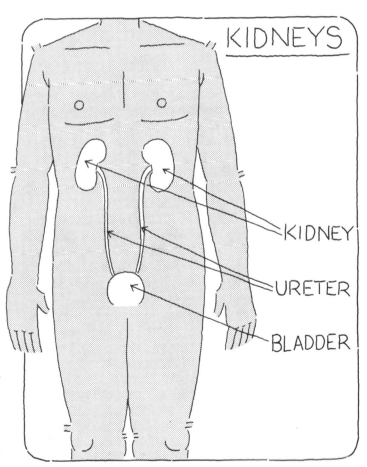

However, there is some risk that the transplant will not work. The body's immune system has a tendency to reject any foreign organs (those that come from someone else), including the kidney. For this reason, the immune systems of both the donor and the recipient are matched very carefully. Also, powerful drugs, called immunosuppressives (see Immuno-

legislator

suppressives), are given to help suppress (hold back) the immune system. Though there are risks, kidney transplantation is highly successful.

Is there anything you can do to prevent kidney disease? It seems that tight control of blood-sugar levels helps prevent kidney disease. Researchers are conducting clinical trials at the Diabetes Control and Complications Trial (see DCCT). One of the things researchers want to find out is the effect that tight diabetes control has on preventing kidney disease. Controlling your blood pressure (see High Blood Pressure) is another preventive measure you can take. Hypertension (high blood pressure) can aggravate any damage to the kidneys. Also, avoiding cigarettes and alcohol, getting adequate sleep, and exercising regularly are all healthy habits that may help you avoid kidney disease.

Until we do find out for sure, remember you are still benefiting from taking control of your diabetes. Don't you feel better since you started controlling your diabetes? Keep up the good work!

legislator
(LEJ-is-LATE-or)

Ever been fed up with Congress? Did you ever try to do something about it? Did you know you could?

So many people fail to pay attention to what our legislators do. Nor do they let their senators and congressional representatives know their views on issues that concern them. That's a shame, considering your legislators are making decisions that do affect you and your quality of living. This includes legislation dealing with diabetes. For example, all government funding that goes toward medical research, including diabetes, is allocated by your legislators.

You need to let your elected officials know how you feel. If you don't let your representatives know your views on an issue, you can't really complain when they don't vote the way you want them to. Your legislators aren't mind readers—let them know how you feel through a letter or a telephone call. Here are some tips for writing your elected officials:

■ Find out who your senators (each state has two) and your representatives (each congressional district has one) are. If you are in doubt, check a copy of the *Almanac of American Politics* or the *Congressional Directory.* Your library should have a copy of one of these. Also, your local American Diabetes Association affiliate or chapter should have a listing of senators and representatives in your state.

■ Specify the topic of concern to you. Don't express multiple topics in one letter. It is better to concentrate on just one issue. If you are concerned about a specific bill, include the name of the bill and its number. (For example: each bill is labeled either "H.R." or "S." before its number. If the bill has "H.R." before its number, this means it was generated in the House of Representatives. An "S." before the number means the bill was generated in the Senate.)

■ Be clear about what you want your legislator to do.

■ Briefly explain the reasons behind your request. Be personal. How would the legislation affect you, your family, your co-workers, or your community?

■ Use your own words instead of using or copying a form letter. Your own words will get read before a form letter will—they also show that you are interested in the issue rather than just following someone else's lead.

■ If you hand-write your letter, be sure it is legible. If you want a reply, ask for one. Be sure to include your name and address at the bottom of the letter.

■ Be timely. Get your letter in the mail before the legislation gets considered.

■ If you get a reply, it may be a form letter. Form letters are not all bad. They usually can give you an indication of the legislator's position on the issue. If the letter is not clear, don't be afraid to write again to ask for clarification. Remember, your legislator works *for you*—and has to answer *to you*.

loneliness
(LONE-lee-ness)

Anyone who has ever been lonely—and virtually every person has—knows that loneliness can go far beyond the presence or absence of other people. You can feel lonely in a crowd, and even, at times, with friends or family.

Social research has found that more and more people are lonely and that such factors as success or where you live— city or country—have little to do with it. More relevant is the depth of our connections to other people and how much time and energy we spend on maintaining relationships.

Many factors can threaten relationships, including illness. When you are hit with an "invisible" chronic disease such as diabetes, which can affect every aspect of your life, a tendency to loneliness can become exaggerated. Upon diagnosis, many people with diabetes later report that they felt "alone" or "lonely." Some believe that other people cannot possibly understand what they are feeling. Others fear that even long-time companions will be less accepting of them now that they have diabetes.

When you feel different from those around you and are afraid of rejection, loneliness may seem preferable to being hurt. It's easy to put up protective walls around yourself and keep other people outside. But don't do it! Loneliness isn't good for you. It's been linked to a variety of illnesses, including migraine headaches, hypertension, and heart disease. In fact, establishing meaningful relationships with others is now seen as a primary factor in a long life.

Fighting loneliness can be hard, but the results are almost always positive. A first step is to reconnect with those important to you. Talk about your diabetes. Let everyone, you and your loved ones, discuss how they feel about the disease. The feelings will probably be strong and include some negative ones. Let them out. Be accepting: Everyone has a right to his or her feelings. Realize that you haven't changed as a human being. And ask for help in coping with diabetes. You will probably be warmly surprised by the supportive response of those who care.

Sometimes, however, you or your family may need profes-

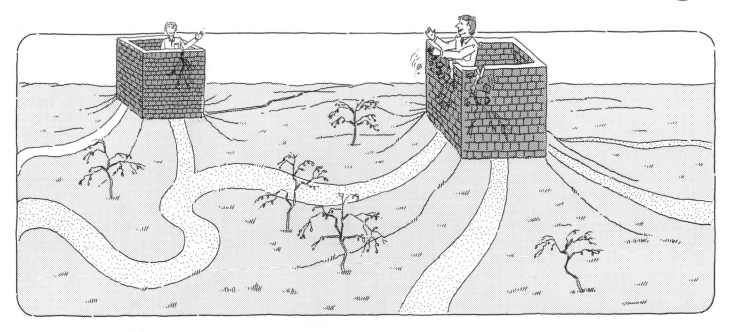

sional guidance to help you get through turbulent times. Your physician can probably recommend a psychotherapist who can help you deal more effectively with the problem. You may find a support group of people who have diabetes particularly helpful. Contact your local American Diabetes Association affiliate for information on one in your area. You may also consider joining a club or a church group.

Finally, you may find having a pet will help cure your loneliness. While involvement with an animal should not substitute for human relationships, the mutual love and caring are very real and beneficial.

macrovascular
(MAK-row-VAS-ku-ler)

Macro means large. And macrovascular refers to large blood vessels (arteries). These arteries are the major "highways" that run throughout your body. They cover long distances and carry large volumes of important products (such as food, oxygen, and nutrients) from the heart to the many "branches" or "side streets" in your body (see Microvascular). For example, one major "highway" would be the vessels in your leg and the "side streets" would be those in your toes.

Like traffic, blood can flow smoothly along unless the "road" gets blocked or congested. This blockage happens when cholesterol, calcium, and fat build up on the inner wall of an artery (see Atherosclerosis). When these major "highways" are blocked, the flow of blood to the "side streets" is limited. When blood flow is decreased, the body parts served by the smaller blood vessels don't get the nourishment they need.

A clogged artery can cause serious problems: clogged arteries of the head can cause a stroke; clogged arteries leading to the heart could cause pain and possibly a heart attack; and clogged arteries in the legs could cause pain and

possibly result in amputation. You need to do what you can to prevent fatty deposits from building up on the walls of your arteries. You are the "traffic cop" and are responsible for keeping these "roads" clear. Keep your diabetes in control, exercise regularly, and limit your intake of cholesterol and fats. The more you work at it, the better the chances that it will be smooth sailin' from head to toe.

marriage
(MARE-ij)

Marriage is a challenge whether you have diabetes or not. Regardless of how compatible you two may be, you likely will have difficulties. You both will bring habits or characteristics into the marriage that will take the other time to get used to. Problems will arise that will put stress on your marriage. Diabetes, too, can be a big challenge in a marriage.

Diabetes can be scary—but don't withdraw from your partner and be afraid by yourself. Coming together and working together as a couple can strengthen your marriage instead of destroying it.

Certainly, those who treat diabetes have seen a great deal of frustration and anger, disaster and divorce. But who's to say diabetes was to blame—it's hard to know whether the same result would have occurred if some other type of major stress had hit these couples.

Anyway, you're lucky. We now know more about diabetes than we ever have and taking control of it has become easier. A better understanding of diabetes will help you handle it—and your marriage—better.

Knowledge is one of the keys to a successful marriage. Both husband and wife need access to current information on diabetes, and peer support to cope with problems as they arise. Having a good understanding of the different aspects of diabetes will help the non-diabetic spouse recognize when diabetes is out of control and needs attending to. Knowledge

meal planning

will help you keep a balance in your life. It will help you keep your sense of humor and the lines of communication open.

It is essential to be continuously open to change and growth. Just as in any marriage, problems don't always get solved "once and for all." Problems can resurface and trouble a marriage in different ways. As the couple grows older and takes on new roles, such as parenting or changing careers, new stresses will evolve. You have to keep working at your marriage and resolving new conflicts. This is a sign not of failure, but of growth!

Couples may need to learn to break some of the traditions that surround marriage. For example, some traditional gender roles, such as cooking or shopping, may need to be negotiated. Perhaps the wife who has diabetes can't stand to be around all the food during preparation. Or the reverse may be true. The husband with diabetes may want to play a more significant role by participating in meal preparation.

While the burden of the disease may seem to fall on the spouse with diabetes alone, the partner who does not have diabetes faces extra stress, too—in addition to worrying about the complications of diabetes. Being a supportive partner to a person with diabetes can be tough. Should you remind the partner to take medications? Should you review the buffet selection and comment on good food choices? Treading the fine line between being supportive and being a pest isn't easy.

Again, these are problems that you have to discuss with one another. You may find you need to renegotiate periodically. A problem "solved" in January may well resurface in a new form by June. Couples who are open in their communication—who can talk honestly about their fears and hopes, wants and needs, angers and joys—have the best chance for a successful marriage.

meal planning
(MEAL PLAN-ing)

One of the great myths of diabetes is that you cannot enjoy good food. True, your choices may be limited a bit, but basically, you can enjoy almost any kind of food. You just need to follow a meal plan. In fact, all people could benefit from following the meal plans designed for people with diabetes.

Of course, having diabetes means you need to strictly limit concentrated sugars in your diet. That's because these cause a rapid rise in blood glucose. Some people will need to limit fats, and still others will need to limit the amount of salt they eat. Other things are important, too. For example, your daily food intake should include some of each nutrient: proteins, carbohydrates, fats, vitamins, and minerals. Your meal plan will make sure you get the right amount of these nutrients to meet your body's needs.

If you take insulin, several things are necessary to keep *your* diabetes under control: You need to properly time meals, snacks, and exercise to match the action of insulin. Also, you need to maintain day-to-day consistency in the amount of carbohydrate, protein, and fat in your diet. These factors all

help make your insulin work more efficiently.

For overweight people with type II diabetes, one of the most important treatments is losing weight. This is often done by limiting calories and increasing exercise under the supervision of a doctor and a dietitian.

The important thing to remember is that your meal plan is individual. You and your doctor or diet counselor will prescribe a meal plan that fits *your* needs. It should provide

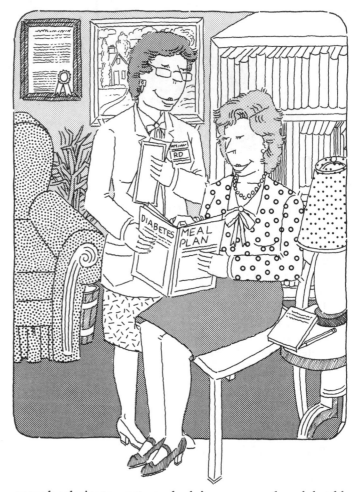

enough calories to meet your body's energy needs and should include foods that you enjoy and find satisfying. The American Diabetes Association recommends that 55 to 60 percent of total daily calories should come from carbohydrates (mainly complex carbohydrates), 12 to 20 percent from protein, and less than 30 percent from fat. For meal planning within these guidelines, try one of the *Month of Meals* menu books available from the ADA. In each one, you'll find an entire month's menus for breakfast, lunch, and dinner, all guaranteed to be healthy and delicious.

meat/meat substitute exchange list
(MEAT SUB-stah-TOOT eks-CHANJ LIST)

Sure, you expect to see prime rib or hamburger on this list. But did you think of such things as squirrel or tofu? Well, they are there, along with peanut butter and bratwurst.

The list is broken down into three categories: lean, medium-fat, and high-fat meat and meat substitutes. When choosing from these lists, you are better off choosing from those items on the lean and medium-fat lists. The choices on these two lists are better for you in terms of helping you decrease your risk for heart disease. The high-fat items are high in cholestrol, saturated fat, and calories.

Also, you should avoid frying foods in deep fat—frying just adds extra fat to your meal. Also, try to trim off any visible fat from the meat before and after preparing it.

Well, we've given you a taste of the Meat exchange list—get a copy of the full exchange list from your American Diabetes Association affiliate and get cooking.

microvascular
(MI-kro-VAS-ku-ler)

The term microvascular refers to the small blood vessels (capillaries) in your body. The capillaries are the "side streets" in your body that branch off from the major "highways" or large blood vessels (see Macrovascular). Some of these "side streets" are in such places as your fingers, toes, kidneys, and eyes.

The capillaries have walls so thin that oxygen and glucose can pass through them and enter the cells. Sometimes, in people with diabetes, the inner lining of these small blood vessels becomes thick and weak. This weakness lets them bleed, leak protein, and decrease the flow of blood through critical tissues, such as those of the kidney.

When blood flow is restricted, the cells do not receive the nutrients they need and may become damaged. For example, if this were to happen to your eye, it may restrict your vision (see Retinopathy). The function of your kidneys, which are nourished by these vessels, can also be affected by damaged capillaries (see Kidneys).

Scientists don't fully understand what causes the capillaries to weaken and become damaged, but they suspect that abnormally high blood-sugar levels are at least partly to blame. These elevated blood-sugar levels deprive critical tissues of essential chemicals that are used for growth and normal function.

Fortunately, it appears that small blood vessel disease can be prevented or at least delayed through proper diabetes control. Along with control, regular checkups with your doctor and eye doctor are necessary to catch problems in their early stages so small problems don't become big ones.

milk exchange list
(MILK eks-CHANJ LIST)

This is the shortest of all the lists. On it you will find all types of milk: whole, lowfat, skim, evaporated, and even lowfat buttermilk. Yogurt is on the list, too. Look for cheeses, however, on the Meat and substitutes list.

Generally, one exchange equals one cup of milk. Eight ounces of yogurt will give you an exchange. Both yogurt and milk are good sources of calcium and protein which are needed for growth and repair of bones. So, be sure to check the Milk Exchange list, drink some milk, and give your bones a break . . . rather, keep your bones from breaking.

miracle cures
(MIR-ah-kal KYERZ)

What do blueberry tea, mineral water, garlic, vitamins, Jerusalem artichokes, and lecithin all have in common? At one time or another, they have all been touted as "miracle cures" for diabetes. Unfortunately, while some of these substances may be part of a good diet, none can cure diabetes.

Some people have claimed, for example, that Jerusalem artichokes contain insulin. Even if this were true—and it isn't—insulin would be broken down in the stomach before it could reach the bloodstream. Jerusalem artichokes do contain a nutrient called *inulin* (a substance similar to fructose), not insulin.

Miracle treatments are common, too. Some chiropractors, for instance, claim that diabetes can be cured by relieving pressure on the spine. To the degree that people—especially those with type I diabetes—avoid proper therapy because of such claims, these treatments can be dangerous. Be wary of wild claims, fad diets, and easy cures. Only change your meal plan or medication schedule in cooperation with an established health professional.

money savers
(MUN-ee SAV-ers)

There's no way to get around it—diabetes is expensive. While your health must come first, it sure doesn't hurt to save some money. Here are a few ideas for making the costs a little more bearable:

■ Buy fresh, unpackaged food instead of processed foods. In addition to being cheaper, they are generally better for you.

■ Buy food in bulk quantities, cook larger batches, and freeze the leftovers.

■ Pool your money with other people who have diabetes and buy supplies wholesale. Use the same co-op idea to buy bulk foods.

■ Do some comparison shopping with mail-order "discount pharmacies."

■ Some people achieve savings by reusing disposable syringes. Manufacturers do not recommend this practice because it increases your risk of infection. Talk to your physician if you are thinking about reusing your syringes.

nephropathy

■ Of course, one of the best ways to cut down on medical expenses is to keep your diabetes under good control. By keeping yourself healthy, you'll keep yourself out of the hospital, and hospitalization is the biggest expense of all.

nephropathy

(ne-FROP-ah-thee)

See Kidneys

neuropathy

(nerr-OP-ah-thee)

A complication of diabetes is diabetic neuropathy—damage to nerves in your body. The most common type is peripheral neuropathy. Peripheral nerves are those nerves that extend outside the brain and spinal cord. (For example, the nerves in your arms and legs.) There are three types of peripheral nerves: motor, sensory, and autonomic.

Your motor nerves are the ones that carry signals to your muscles to tell them to move. They help you to do things like walk or move your fingers and toes. Sensory nerves help you to sense things—warmth, coolness, texture, shape, movement, and pain. The autonomic nerves work to help regulate such things as the pace of your heartbeats, your blood pressure, and sweating. They also help carry out the function of your intestinal tract, bladder, and sex organs.

Damage to any one of these nerves means damage to the functions they carry out. For instance, if the motor nerve fibers are damaged, your muscles may be weakened. For people with diabetes, the muscles that control eye movement are most often affected. Or you could suffer from a burning sensation in your legs when you move them.

If damage occurs to the sensory nerves, you may lose feeling in a part of your body such as your foot. You may not be able to sense a rock inside your shoe or feel the hot sand at the beach. Even worse, you may not feel a puncture wound. If left untreated, the wound could become infected. In other people, walking can become difficult and painful.

Impairment of the autonomic nerves may weaken the effectiveness of your digestive tract. If the small intestine is affected, you may get diarrhea. (When this happens, the diarrhea generally occurs at night.) Paralysis of the bladder is another complication of autonomic neuropathy. This causes urine to remain in the bladder, and must be treated to avoid infection. Also, this type of neuropathy could make you impotent (see Impotence).

Cases of neuropathy range from mild to severe. But it is rarely fatal and many times the symptoms last only a few months and then disappear. What can you do to prevent neuropathy? Studies are still going on to determine what you can do to prevent this complication. Your best bet is to keep diabetes in control. You also need to keep in touch with your doctor through regular checkups. This will help you catch complications before they get worse.

So far, there is no specific treatment for neuropathy. However, good control of diabetes appears to help. In addition, you need to be careful to head off further complications and avoid injuries. For example, if you lose feeling in your feet, you will want to inspect them daily to be sure that they are not injured. Inspecting your feet daily will help you ward off infections before they get out of hand. (See Foot Care.)

Neuropathy is an unpleasant fact among those with diabetes, but it doesn't have to happen to you. While there are no guarantees that you won't experience some form of neuropathy, do all you can to avoid it through proper diabetes management.

nonobese type II

(non-o-bees TIPE TWO)

Ever hear that only obese people have type II diabetes? But you're thin and you have type II? Why is this so?

Some people are not actually overweight, but their bodies act as if they were. These individuals appear to be thin but actually have more body fat than muscle. Technically, they are overweight and their bodies act as if they were obese. You may fall into this category and might need to follow a regimen similar to that which an obese person with type II diabetes would.

Everyone with type II diabetes needs to control his or her diabetes through meal planning and exercise. Also, many lean people with type II diabetes are also treated with insulin injections. Treatment for some people may also include oral medication.

For anyone who has diabetes, exercise is advisable. Regular moderate exercise, such as running or swimming laps, helps to decrease fat and increase muscle. These changes, as well as the exercise itself, appear to improve the body's ability to use insulin. Another bonus of exercise is that it helps to keep your weight down. If you plan to start an exercise program, check with your doctor first.

You will also need to test your blood regularly to monitor your control (see Blood Tests). Because type II diabetes is generally more stable than type I (insulin-dependent) diabetes, you can probably test blood less often than a person with type I. Check with your doctor to find what would be best for you.

The cause behind type II diabetes in lean people is not known. Most people with type II have high blood sugar because they have the dual problem of an insulin shortage and insulin resistance (see Insulin Resistance). That is, the pancreas does not produce enough insulin for the body's needs, and the cells elsewhere in the body do not use insulin efficiently.

Remember that treatment plans are meant to be fine-tuned occasionally to meet your changing lifestyle needs. Your doctor can help you make these adjustments as you need them.

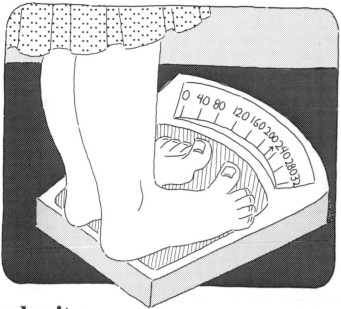

obesity

(o-BEES-i-tee)

One of the fastest-growing chronic diseases today, obesity affects millions of Americans. Any person whose weight is 20 percent over normal is considered obese. However, your weight could fall within what might be considered normal and you still could be obese. When body fat exceeds the amount of muscle, obesity exists, even though actual weight is within the normal range. The causes of obesity can be social, economic, cultural, and psychological. The tendency for obesity runs in families.

Most weight is gained gradually over a period of years, accumulating almost unnoticed. Extra pounds can creep up on you. Did you know that by eating a single slice of bread more than you need each day, you can add 7.3 pounds in a year? In 10 years that's 73 pounds! Eating habits formed early in childhood are usually followed throughout life. Ideally, the amount of calories people eat should decrease with age and diminished activity. Unfortunately, many people are obese because they eat too much and exercise too little.

What role does obesity play in people with diabetes? Obesity seems to cause insulin receptors to shut down or become resistant to insulin's action. In other words, the body produces enough insulin, but the body does not fully accept the action of that insulin. Our bodies have receptors (see Receptors) that "grab" the insulin as it flows through the blood and deliver it to the cells.

To make up for insulin resistance, the beta cells (the insulin producers) of the pancreas work harder and make extra insulin. That's why many obese people do not develop type II diabetes in their younger years. However, years later the beta cells may slow down and not produce enough insulin to meet the body's needs. Without the extra insulin, glucose then piles up in the blood. The result: diabetes. As the obesity continues, the diabetes gets worse.

If you develop type II diabetes, your doctor will likely work with you to help you lose weight. For many people, weight loss is instrumental in making type II diabetes disappear.

Basically, if you have type II diabetes, you will need to exercise and follow a meal plan.

We know that exercising and dieting are tough. But we also know they are well worth it. You'll probably feel—and be—a lot healthier.

ophthalmologist

(OFF-thal-MALL-ah-jist)

An ophthalmologist is a physician (M.D.) who specializes in diagnosing and treating eye disorders. He or she also performs surgery and prescribes glasses and medication. (An *ophthalmologist* is not the same as an *optometrist*. See Optometrist.)

If you have diabetes, you are at risk for developing eye disorders (see Retinopathy). It is important that you catch problems early so they can be treated. For this reason, we recommend that you have an ophthalmic exam at least once a year. The earlier these problems are detected, the better your chances they can be corrected.

optician

(op-tish-an)

An optician is the person who adjusts the frames to your eyeglasses and grinds the lenses to fit the frames. *An optician is not a medical physician and cannot diagnose or treat eye problems.* (See Ophthalmologist.)

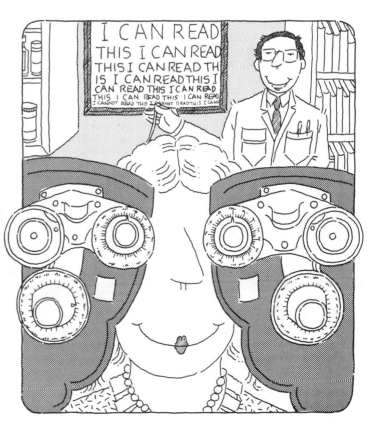

optometrist

(op-TOM-ah-trist)

Many people go to an optometrist to have an eye exam and to get a prescription for glasses. An optometrist can test your vision to see if you are having problems in refraction (how well your eyes focus), such as farsightedness or nearsightedness.

Once your optometrist has assessed your problem, he or she can prescribe glasses. An optometrist can also diagnose eye problems. An optometrist is not a medical physician and cannot prescribe medication needed to treat diseases of the eye. Nor can an optometrist perform eye surgery. (See Ophthalmologist.)

oral agents

(OR-al A-jent)

Do you ever wish there was a pill that could make your diabetes disappear? We wish it were so, too. The closest thing we have to it is good diabetes control—exercise, meal planning, and insulin or oral medication. We have discussed the first three topics elsewhere in this publication. Now it's time we talk about oral agents.

What are oral agents? Properly, they are called oral hypoglycemic agents. Remember the word hypoglycemic? It means low blood sugar and oral hypoglycemic agents are designed to do just that—lower your blood sugar. If you have insulin-dependent (type I) diabetes, you won't benefit from oral agents. Only people with non-insulin-dependent (type II) diabetes can use oral agents. But oral agents are no substitute for proper meal planning and exercise. These two (exercise and meal planning) alone are the *very* best treatment for type II diabetes. By themselves, they can often bring blood-glucose levels down to normal. However, if you have made a serious attempt to lower your blood-glucose level and it still remains high, you may want to supplement your meal and exercise regimen with an oral agent.

It is not completely understood how oral agents work. Some people with type II diabetes apparently don't make enough insulin for their body's needs. For others it seems the cells in their bodies aren't receptive to the insulin produced. (See Insulin Resistance, Receptors.) Some people have both problems. Oral agents seem to improve both problems—they improve the production of insulin by the pancreas and help make the body cells more receptive to insulin.

Oral agents don't work for everyone with type II diabetes. The agents may lower blood sugar a little, but this may not be enough. And oral agents sometimes quit working after a period of months or years. So, don't expect oral agents to be a miracle cure to high blood sugar—they aren't.

If your doctor has decided to put you on an oral agent, be sure to use common sense and use the drug properly. In general, oral agents are safe, but like other drugs, you need to use them carefully. Some people do have reactions to oral agents, such as skin rashes, upset stomach, and a flushing of the skin while consuming alcohol. Always report any changes, such as an allergic reaction, to your doctor. Any problem may be minor, but it is best to check with your doctor just in case.

Some people, especially those who are older, eat poorly, or have impaired liver or kidney function, may develop severe hypoglycemia (low blood glucose). This condition is difficult to reverse and requires emergency treatment (see Hypoglycemia). What makes this condition particularly serious is that it can be confused with a stroke, so treatment may be delayed. And a delay in treatment could cause brain damage.

If you are using oral agents and decide you would like to consider controlling diabetes with just weight control and exercise, see your doctor. *Do not* stop taking your medicine on your own. The consequences of having no medicine and no medical supervision may well be worse than any harm the pills may do. Also, don't forget to test your blood regularly to be sure your blood-glucose levels are as near to normal as possible.

Again, oral agents are not miracle drugs—they may work for you and they may not. And they don't replace the best method of control for you—meal planning and exercise.

pancreas

(PAN-kree-us)

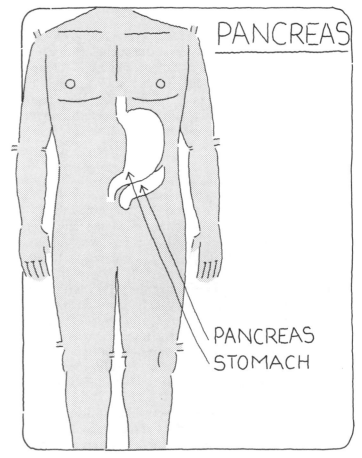

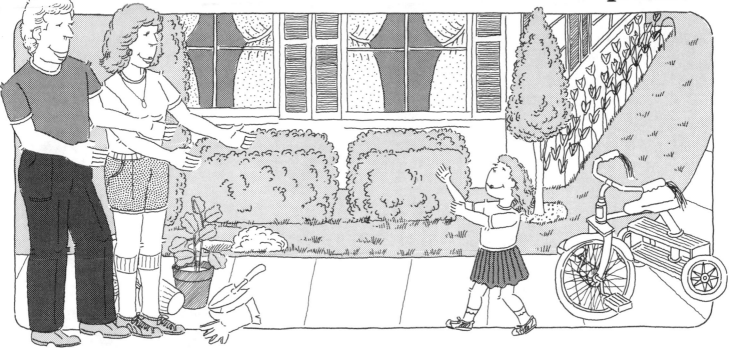

This comma-shaped gland, about six inches in length and located just behind the stomach, has two big jobs. First, it produces enzymes for digesting food. Second, the pancreas produces hormones that regulate the use of fuels (mainly glucose and fat) by the body. This second role of the pancreas, known as the *endocrine* function, is what fails to work in people with type I diabetes and, in many cases, those with type II diabetes. Specifically, the pancreas doesn't produce enough insulin, and in the case of type I diabetes, virtually stops producing insulin.

When the pancreas is working normally, glucose enters the blood and flows through the *islets of Langerhans*, masses of cells sprinkled throughout the pancreas. These islets release insulin into the blood. Insulin permits glucose to enter body cells, either to be burned immediately for energy or stored for later use.

A second hormone secreted by the pancreas, glucagon, keeps the action of insulin in check. Instead of lowering blood sugar, glucagon *raises* it, by breaking down a starch called glycogen, which is stored in the liver, into glucose. Glucagon is secreted when blood-glucose levels are lower than what the body needs. That is why glucagon injections can be used to treat insulin reactions.

parents

(PEAR-ent)

Raising a child who has diabetes can pose special challenges to parents. But if your expectations for your child are reasonable and you are supportive and encourage two-way communication, you are on the right track to helping your child grow into a healthy, independent, and mature adult.

Here are some helpful suggestions:

■ If you are overly anxious, seek help in calming down. Your child may pick up on your feelings and worry too.

■ Discuss with your doctor the tasks your child can reasonably be expected to handle. Remember that age and maturity level count a lot. Also, try to set realistic targets for blood-sugar control and work toward keeping control as tight as possible without making your child overly nervous.

■ Try to bring out your child's feelings—and let him or her know you understand. For instance, if the child becomes upset at injection time, you can try helping him or her know you understand his or her concerns about taking injections. It won't help make your child like injections any more, but it may help him or her feel happier knowing that you care.

■ Be supportive without hovering. Drawing the line is not easy, but an example would be helping the child with an injection now and then. But don't help every time. If, for instance, the child is ill, your giving the shot gives him or her the message that you are there for backup when the going gets rough. Of course, a four-year-old could not be expected to give his or her own shots.

■ If you need help coping, consider talking to other parents who you feel have raised a child with diabetes well. You might want to attend a group for parents at your local American Diabetes Association chapter. You might consider seeking the help of a family therapist or other counselor, or talking to a physician, nurse, or diabetes educator familiar with diabetes in children and adolescents.

Parenting is never an easy job, and when your child has diabetes, you need all the help and support you can get.

potatoes

(pah-TATE-ohs)

The poor potato has been given a bad name—no, we're not referring to the name "spud." Back in the 16th century, it was blamed for causing illnesses from leprosy to syphilis. Today,

pregnancy

the potato has been shunned by many a dieter who has mistakenly accused it of being fattening. Not so—it's not the potato that heaps on the calories. It's the stuff you put on top of it!

All by itself, butter or margarine on a spud can *double* your calories. A plain, medium potato is about 100 calories—and so is a tablespoon of butter or margarine. But, unlike butter, your naked potato, which is composed mostly of complex carbohydrate (starch), gives you vitamin C and many B vitamins, as well as some high-quality protein, fiber, and iron. Avoid peeling potatoes, though, because you peel away a lot of nutrients by removing the skin.

Instead of butter, margarine, or sour cream, consider topping your potato with cottage cheese (17 calories per tablespoon), plain yogurt (8 calories per tablespoon), or herbs and spices (no calories).

See, the potato isn't so bad. Now, go spread the word, but remember not to spread the butter.

pregnancy
(PREG-nan-see)

Thinking of having a baby? Are you worried that your baby won't be healthy or normal? And are you wondering how a pregnancy will affect your diabetes?

Well, relax—it's normal to be worried about pregnancy and about how the baby will turn out. You know what? That's part of being a parent. Everyone worries about these things. Of course, there was a time when those with diabetes had several things to worry about. Having a baby posed a definite risk. However, doctors have vastly increased the odds for diabetic women to have healthy babies.

The key to this success has been the realization that *excellent diabetes control before conception and then throughout pregnancy* is vital to the health of the baby. So, if you're thinking about having a baby, get your diabetes in control first. The first weeks of development are very important for your baby. Most birth defects occur when the baby's organs are forming (within the first weeks after conception). Many women don't realize they are pregnant during this time and don't take proper precautions.

What should you do to keep your diabetes in control during pregnancy? The same things you do to keep your diabetes in control during regular times: proper meal planning and exercise. In addition, you may need to test your blood more frequently than you normally do to closely track your blood-glucose levels. While insulin can't be passed on to your baby, blood glucose can. When your blood glucose rises, so does your baby's. The high blood sugar will cause your baby's pancreas to produce excessive insulin. Too much insulin will cause your baby to become larger than normal. By keeping your diabetes in control, you can keep your baby down to a normal size.

A normal pregnancy lasts nine months, or 40 weeks. The pregnancy is divided into three three-month periods of time called *trimesters*. Let's go through the different stages of pregnancy to give you an idea of what you and your baby will go through:

■ The first trimester. This is a time for you to store nutrients, mainly fat. The fetus grows slowly. If your diabetes was a challenge to control before pregnancy, you may have even more trouble with high and low blood sugars. You'll need to work closely with your doctor and dietitian to meet these challenges.

You may well be given a meal plan high in calories, especially protein for building tissues. *Do not try to lose weight during pregnancy*—you will underfeed your baby.

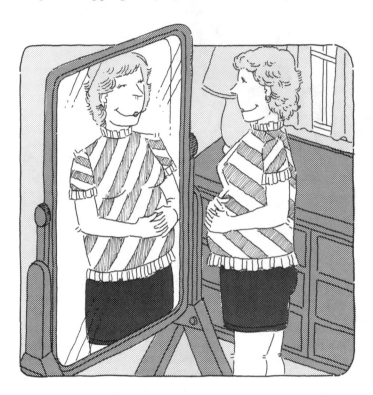

You will need an initial exam by an obstetrician (a medical doctor who specializes in childbirth), with follow-ups every few weeks. You will also need to have your eyes and kidneys evaluated periodically, so that any needed treatment can be started promptly.

■ The second trimester. In the later part of this trimester, your baby grows dramatically, and the *placenta* will pour out hormones. (The placenta is the material which surrounds the baby in the mother's uterus. Nutrients pass through it from mother to baby.) As a result, your blood sugar may soar, and you may well need two to three times more insulin than you normally take. Don't worry. Your diabetes is not getting worse. The extra demand for insulin occurs in all pregnant women at this time. (Sometimes in a woman who doesn't have diabetes, the pancreas can't handle the additional demand for insulin, and she will temporarily have diabetes. See Gestational Diabetes.) Again, to ensure good control, you will have to test often and, in response, adjust your food, insulin, or exercise as directed by your doctor.

By the end of this trimester, you will be seeing your obstetrician once a week and may be in daily contact with your diabetologist. A sonogram (ultrasound) and other tests of the baby's progress may be done.

■ The third trimester. At about your eighth month, your insulin requirement should level off. Your weekly visits to the obstetrician might now be supplemented with special tests such as a sonogram to monitor your baby's progress and to determine when the baby should be delivered.

All diabetic women used to be delivered early—around the 37th, rather than the 40th, week of pregnancy. But now many obstetricians are able to decide case-by-case whether a woman will be able to carry to term (the full nine months) or close to it. The decision depends, in part, on your health and control and the baby's health and size. If your diabetes control has been less than perfect, the baby may be oversized, and may need to be delivered earlier. Depending on your health and the health and progress of your baby, you may have to have a Caesarean section (C-section). A C-section is a surgical operation for delivering a baby. It is done by cutting through the walls of the mother's abdomen and uterine wall to where the baby is. The baby is lifted out of the abdominal area.

Whew! We got you through the nine months of pregnancy and you have a beautiful, healthy baby. Now, if you think the nine months were tough, remember you've now got some 20 years of parenting ahead of you. But cheer up—maybe there will be a cure to those dreadful teens by the time your little darling hits adolescence.

pumps
(PUMPS)

You want tight control of your diabetes but you can't stand to give yourself injections several times a day. What are you going to do? You might want to try an insulin pump.

What's an insulin pump? It is essentially a mechanical syringe that stays attached to a person round-the-clock. Instead of separate shots, the pump gives continuous drips of insulin throughout the day (called the *basal* infusion). Before meals, the person presses a button on the pump to get an extra squirt (called a *bolus*) of insulin to counter the blood-glucose surge that will result from the food.

Because insulin needs vary, the basal and bolus doses are carefully determined by the pump-user's physician. Adjustments must be made by the user in response to frequent (four to six times a day) daily home blood tests. If you were to get a pump, your doctor would probably calculate your proper basal level. He would also give you some general guidelines for adjusting the bolus level to compensate for food, exercise, and the results of self-monitoring of blood glucose. An insulin pump is not an artificial pancreas. For this reason, frequent blood-glucose monitoring is *essential*.

Insulin pumps are not for everybody. The best candidates are those insulin-users who cannot achieve good control any other way, including multiple injections (four or more shots a day). Other good candidates can include pregnant women (who need to maintain tight control for the health of their baby) and highly motivated people who show a strong willingness, and the ability, to make insulin pump therapy work for them.

Insulin pumps are generally worn at a person's side on a belt. The pumps are about the size and shape of a "beeper," and the trend is to make them even smaller. The insulin stored in the pump passes through a tube into a needle inserted under the skin, usually in the abdomen.

Among the advantages of pump therapy, as voiced by pump users and their physicians, are:
■ The good feeling and added energy that accompany good control.
■ The possibility that tight control will help prevent, or slow the development of, long-term complications. (See DCCT.)
■ The flexibility provided by using only Regular (short-acting) insulin. Because a person does not have to time meals to meet the peaking action of a shot of slow-acting insulin, meals can be delayed fairly easily when necessary. And because it is easier to predict how short-acting insulin will enter the bloodstream, there may be less guesswork in fine-tuning insulin doses to keep blood glucose normal.

However (You knew this was coming, didn't you?), there are some disadvantages to using insulin pumps. You should weigh these disadvantages carefully, and discuss them with your physician, before deciding to use a pump:
■ The possibility of severe insulin reactions, especially if the user does not test frequently enough or does not properly adjust insulin dosage, food, and exercise in response to the tests. In particular, the basal rate must be very carefully set to avoid insulin reactions around 3 a.m., when blood sugar is naturally at its lowest.
■ The possibility (although unlikely) of mechanical problems or of the needle becoming dislodged without a person realizing it. Because only small amounts of short-acting insulin are used in the pump, blood glucose can soar quickly if the pump is accidentally disconnected.
■ Local skin irritation. This is the most common problem with pumps. Often it is caused by the tape used to secure the needle, but it can also be caused by allergies to metal needles or to the kind of insulin used. A more serious problem is infection. Some people who have had frequent infections at the insertion site have had to stop using the pump.
■ The adjustments necessary to work the insulin pump into a person's daily life. Bathing, sleeping, and dressing are just a few of the daily routines that have to be changed to accommodate an insulin pump. Of course, people vary greatly in what they consider inconveniences.

So, there you have it—the pump. It may be for you. If you think so, discuss the possibility with your doctor. If not, flip back to the "I's" and read the section on injections.

questions
(KWES-chahns)

There is no such thing as a foolish question—it is only foolish not to ask. Even your doctor had to learn by asking questions. You should never feel embarrassed to ask basic questions of your doctor or of other health professionals. And you should choose a doctor who will take the time to explain diabetes to you, and who respects your desire to know.

rebound

(REE-bownd)

Ever hear of someone marrying on the rebound? Well, if you overhear a friend who has diabetes talking about "rebound," don't jump to conclusions—he or she may be talking about a problem of diabetes that generally happens because of poor diabetes management.

Rebound is known as the *Somogyi effect*, named after Dr. Michael Somogyi, who first identified the problem. Rebound is an abnormally high rise in your blood sugar after an episode of low blood sugar. It often happens like this: You take too much insulin, exercise too hard, or eat too little and have an insulin reaction (low blood sugar) as a result. But for some reason (perhaps you are asleep), you don't realize you are having a reaction and, therefore, you fail to treat it. So, your blood sugar continues to fall, and drops so low that your emergency system goes into gear. It pours out hormones to raise blood sugar and works so hard it overcompensates. In addition, by this time, your blood insulin level may be falling. So, your blood sugar actually soars (the "rebound"), like a ball that bounces after having been thrown against the floor.

The next time you test your blood, you see that your blood sugar is high. So, what do you do? Give yourself extra insulin, and in the process, cause a vicious cycle of insulin reaction, leading to high blood sugar, leading to taking too much insulin, leading again to an insulin reaction.

Any of the following signs may indicate a rebound problem:

■ reactions that cannot be explained by unusual exercise or skipping food
■ constant hunger, often with weight gain
■ waking in the morning with headaches, sweats, or chills
■ moodiness at the same time of day each day
■ nightmares or night terrors
■ worsening of diabetes symptoms, instead of improvement, when insulin dose is raised
■ wide variations in blood and/or urine sugar
■ frequent ketones in the urine, especially overnight

If you have any of these problems, contact your doctor. If you do suffer from rebound, your doctor should be able to adjust the amount or timing of the insulin you take, and may ask you to do some blood-sugar readings early in the morning (between 2 a.m. and 4 a.m.). (Sometimes rebound is confused with dawn phenomenon. See Dawn Phenomenon.)

receptors

(re-SEP-tors)

In recent years, *receptors* have been linked to many diseases. Receptors are substances that sit on the surface of a cell. In diabetes, the receptor problem occurs in many people with non-insulin-dependent (type II) diabetes. Normally, for insulin to stimulate the cells to take up glucose from the blood, insulin has to link up with *insulin receptors*. These receptors are like locks or keyholes that only insulin molecules, which act like keys, can fit. We don't know why, but obesity—especially obesity combined with inactivity—causes these insulin receptors to stop working or resist insulin's action. (See Insulin Resistance.) In other words, the lock no longer recognizes the key. The receptors will also shut down if there is too much insulin in the blood. As a result, a lot of the insulin remains outside the cells, and therefore, so does glucose. When the insulin and glucose cannot get into the cells for any reason, including a receptor problem, blood sugar rises.

Fortunately, it appears that for people with type II diabetes, exercise can help correct the body's insensitivity to insulin. Researchers have discovered that some cells respond to insulin better soon after a person has exercised and for several days after. This appears to indicate that regular exercise would help keep a person's body sensitive to insulin all the time.

relaxation

(REE-lak-SAY-shun)

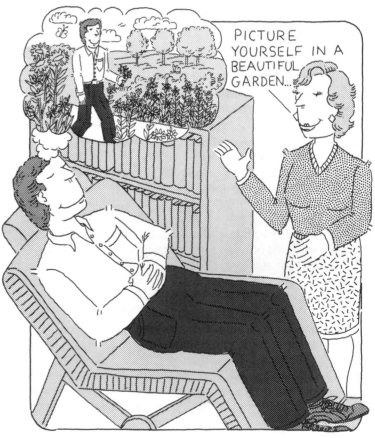

Stress can raise blood sugar, and knowing how to relax yourself can help you to prevent outside stresses from affecting you. Here's a rundown of techniques to help you relax:

In *biofeedback*, you are connected to a monitor. You imagine the effect you want to produce in your body, such as a change in temperature, and the monitor tells you how well your thoughts are controlling your body's reactions.

During *meditation*, you focus your mind on a single image, word, or phrase. Through such focusing, thoughts of daily troubles slip away and you can reach a deep state of relaxation.

In *guided imagery*, a guide helps you imagine yourself in the midst of pleasant scenes, such as walking through a lush garden, smelling the flowers, and feeling the warm sun bathing your body.

In *self-hypnosis*, you direct your body with your thoughts.

In *progressive relaxation*, you tense and relax one set of muscles at a time, working from one part of your body to another.

In *yoga*, you gently stretch your body by performing slow exercise movements and postures.

If you want to try any of these techniques, check with your doctor. Your local American Diabetes Association chapter may also be able to point you to a reputable program.

In a small percentage of people with diabetes, the condition progresses into *proliferative retinopathy*. This occurs when new blood vessels form in and around the retina, branch out or proliferate, and invade other areas of the eye. Scars may also form along these vessels. Eventually, the scar tissue will shrink. When this happens, the scar tissue may pull on the retina and loosen it. If the retina is pulled loose, your vision could be distorted.

Eye doctors can easily diagnose retinopathy using an ophthalmoscope, which gives a magnified view of the inner eye. The best treatment for proliferative retinopathy is a laser technique called *panretinal photocoagulation*, a treatment performed by an ophthalmologist. An intense beam of light is focused on the retina to make many small burns in areas not used for central vision. Performed early enough, this treatment usually causes the abnormal blood vessels to shrink and disappear. Those with moderate to severe proliferative retinopathy may benefit to some degree from photocoagulation. The procedure is usually done right in the ophthalmologist's office.

We've established that you need to keep your blood sugar in control. But in addition, you need an ophthalmic exam at least once a year. Of course, if you have any vision problems, the sooner you visit an eye doctor the better off you will be.

retinopathy

(rhett-in-OP-ah-thee)

While a great number of people with diabetes worry about going blind, only a small percentage ever do. Still, diabetes is the leading cause of non-traumatic blindness (blindness not caused by an injury) among working-age people in the United States. But, those who do develop retinopathy can be treated effectively—if it is caught early.

What is retinopathy? It is an eye disorder. The retina is the area inside the eyeball that receives images of objects and sends information about the images to the brain. Just as diabetes can cause changes in large blood vessels (see Macrovascular) throughout the body, it can also cause tiny bulges in the walls of the small blood vessels (see Microvascular) in the retina. When this happens, fluid may leak from the vessels and build up in the retina, and tiny deposits of fat may form.

When these changes occur and are limited to the retina, the condition is called *background retinopathy*. This is the common, mild form of retinopathy. It does not generally interfere with vision, unless it involves a small area of the eye called the *macula*. The macula is the part of the retina that gives us our sharpest vision. Background retinopathy occurs in at least half of all people with diabetes after they have had diabetes for 10 to 15 years. Background retinopathy normally does not require treatment, although its presence should encourage you to pay especially close attention to diabetes control. The effect of good control on retinopathy that has already gone into the advanced stages is unclear. However, it seems that good control can help prevent retinopathy, or at least slow its progress.

running

(RUNN-ing)

A lot of runners are like fishermen—they have a tendency to fib. While fishermen tell tales about the one that got away, runners tend to stretch the truth a bit on how far they run each day. But that's OK—the important thing is they are exercising. And exercising is one of the keys to good diabetes control.

Since you are concerned about your health and want to keep your diabetes in control, you will want to start an exercise program. Right? Well, running is one option worth looking into. Running gives you an excellent aerobic workout. (An aerobic workout is one that is continuous and rhythmical and stimulates the heart and lungs.) It is inexpensive and you don't have to join a club, nor do you have to travel far to participate.

If you think running might be for you, consult your doctor first. Any exercise program you choose should be approved by your doctor before you start. Then:

■ Begin slowly and gradually increase your level of activity. If you are totally out of shape, a week or more of brisk walking at increasing distances is advisable. Then alternate by running short distances and then walking, and then running a little more. Don't overdo it—you'll be doing yourself more harm than good.

■ Get a good pair of shoes. Running is hard on your body and your feet. You need a pair of shoes that will give you good support and will absorb some of the shock of your body weight bearing down on your legs. Good shoes are a must for runners with diabetes who are prone to foot problems.

■ Run with a friend. You are better off running with someone who knows you have diabetes and can treat you should

school

you have a reaction. If you can't find someone to go with you, at least let someone know your route and when you expect to be back.

■ Be sure to carry some ID that says you have diabetes, states the medication you take, and gives a phone number for prompt help. If you do have a severe reaction, this information will help whoever comes to your aid.

■ To be on the safe side, if you take insulin, always carry some form of concentrated, easily absorbed sugar while running. While many runners with diabetes do not consider hypoglycemia a serious problem, it doesn't make sense to take that risk.

■ As you start your new exercise program, watch carefully for any changes in your diet or medication requirements. Monitor your blood-glucose levels as you increase your level of activity. Discuss any changes with your doctor, who can help you adjust your diabetes regimen.

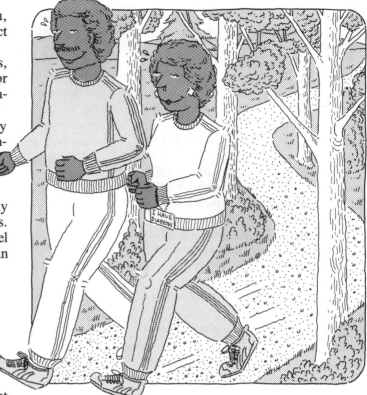

school

(SKOOL)

Remember your first day at a new school? The different surroundings, unfamiliar faces, and the new teacher. That's enough to make your child's first day at school stressful—and if he or she has diabetes, even more so. Well, there is not much you can do about the new environment, but you can help relieve your concerns about diabetes, as well as your son's or daughter's.

How? Here are some helpful steps that may help lessen any anxiety you may have about releasing your budding genius to the world of study:

■ Teach your child as much about diabetes as possible—what to expect and how to cope. The more your child knows about diabetes, the better he or she will become at maintaining good diabetes control on his or her own.

■ Send along quick-energy foods for a snack before gym, and consider sending full lunches because school meals don't always fit with the diabetes meal plan.

■ Educate the school personnel who will have contact with your child (teachers—particularly gym teachers and coaches, the school nurse, and the principal). Try to set up a conference with these key people before school begins. Explain how diabetes affects your youngster. Bring along American

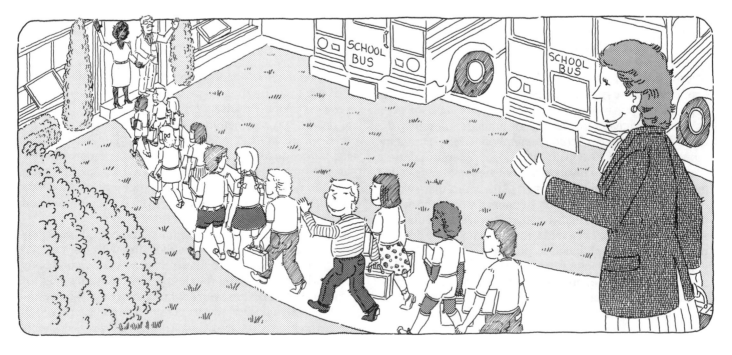

Diabetes Association publications about diabetes, and make sure every adult who sees your son or daughter during the school day has a copy. (The pamphlet *A Word to Teachers and Child-Care Providers* and the booklet *Caring for Children With Diabetes* are two you might consider.) Provide the school nurse with your child's complete medical record. Encourage the teacher to call you when necessary to discuss any concerns. The closer your relationship with the teacher and other school personnel, the more likely they are to be aware of your youngster's special concerns.

■ Be prepared for emergency situations. Make sure the teacher or school nurse has the names and phone numbers of people who can help your child should he or she have an insulin reaction at school. Make sure the teacher or nurse knows how to recognize the signs of an insulin reaction early enough to give your child sugar quickly.

Once you have prepared your child and yourself for all eventualities, let your youngster enjoy school to the fullest and without unnecessary restrictions. These are exciting years of growth and personal discovery, which can be hindered by a parent who is overprotective. Chances of serious trouble are remote if you have followed these guidelines, so learn to let go.

self-monitoring
(SELF-MAWN-ah-tor-ing)

Years ago, getting an accurate measurement of your blood-glucose level required a visit to your doctor or hospital. Now, because *self*-monitoring of blood glucose is possible, *you* can test your blood anytime and anywhere you like.

There are two methods of self-monitoring. One way is through the use of test strips. You prick one of your fingers with a special needle (a lancet), place a drop of blood on the strip, and wait a few minutes. You then compare the color of the strip with the colors on a chart (usually provided with the container that the strips come in). The color chart gives you an approximate reading of what your blood-glucose level is. Another, and more accurate, method of measuring your blood-glucose level is with a glucose meter. Instead of matching the test strip to a chart, you insert the strip in a meter that will ''read'' it for you. Many doctors prefer meters over the visual color chart method because it eliminates any mistakes you may make by improperly matching colors. Technology is moving so rapidly in this arena that soon you may be able to know your blood-glucose level without drawing blood.

Why bother monitoring blood glucose? Self-monitoring of blood glucose allows you to make timely adjustments in food, exercise, and medication. For instance, if you have just finished an exercise routine, your blood-sugar level may be lower than you want it to be. By testing your blood, you may find you need to eat something to raise your blood sugar to a safer level. (Urine tests do not give you an accurate measurement of the amount of glucose in your blood. See Urine Tests.)

People who want to maintain tight control of their diabetes find self-monitoring indespensible. (Tight control means keeping blood sugar at or near normal, or nondiabetic, levels.) Insulin-users following intensive treatment plans (three or more injections a day) frequently test their blood four times a day (at least until they achieve the level of control they desire). Based on the test results, they may adjust their insulin dose or the amount of food they intend to eat, or they exercise a little more or less than planned. All these adjustments are made according to plans worked out *in advance* with their doctors. *Do not* alter your insulin dose without your doctor's guidance.

Anyone with diabetes can benefit from self-monitoring, and especially people who use insulin. The American Diabetes Association strongly urges the following individuals to use self-monitoring of blood glucose:

■ Those who use insulin pumps and those who are taking multiple daily insulin injections with the goal of tight control.

■ Women who are pregnant or those considering pregnancy. Tight control of diabetes before getting pregnant is an important step toward a healthy pregnancy.

■ Those who use insulin and have frequent low blood-sugar episodes. Also, those who have trouble recognizing the warning signs of an insulin reaction.

The American Diabetes Association also encourages the use of self blood-glucose monitoring among the following:

■ Anyone who requires insulin for diabetes treatment.

■ People whose renal thresholds are unusually high or low, making it particularly difficult to gauge blood sugar on the basis of urine tests alone. (The renal threshold is the point at which glucose "spills over" into the urine.)

■ People who need to take unusually large doses of insulin.

■ Any person with diabetes trying to improve his or her blood-glucose control.

If you're thinking about self-monitoring, check with your doctor first. Your doctor or a member of your health-care team will be able to show you how to properly test your blood glucose. You need to do the tests properly to get valid results.

Self-monitoring of blood glucose can be expensive because of the cost of a meter and the test strips. But when you consider the possibility of being and feeling healthier and avoiding complications and medical bills, self-monitoring may be well worth it.

sex
(SEKS)

Do enjoy it! For the person with diabetes, sex offers some extra benefits beyond pleasure. First, it's a great way to relax, and you *know* that reducing stress in your life is important. Second, it's a fantastic form of exercise if you need to lose weight. A lingering, passionate kiss burns up about 12 calories. Depending on the extent of movement, a night of lovemaking can consume from 150 to 300 calories or more. The more active you are, the better. If you enjoy lovemaking after dinner, you also will be helping blunt the typical

sick days

post-meal rise in blood sugar. So carry the candelabra from the dinner table to the bedroom and tell your partner it's "doctor's orders."

Having problems? Yes, diabetes can interfere with your sex life, but fortunately, many problems can be solved through improved diabetes control. For example, women with diabetes are more likely to have vaginal infections. These infections are caused by elevated blood- and urine-sugar levels that allow fungi and bacteria to grow. And the fatigue that accompanies high sugar levels can inhibit interest in *any* "active" work or play, including sex.

More serious are the difficulties caused by diabetic neuropathy (see Neuropathy). Usually, it causes numbness of the feet. Sometimes, though, it also impairs the nerve fibers that affect the pelvic organs. Then, the stimulation system can bog down and sexual arousal fails to occur. In women, the result may be a lack of lubrication and painful intercourse. A simple solution may be an outside source of lubrication (such as K-Y Jelly). In men, erection may be delayed or absent. More intense stimulation or other forms of sexual play are possible alternatives. For those men who, unfortunately, lose the ability to have an erection entirely, a mechanical device that produces an erection may be an option (see Impotence).

If you have a sexual problem, it may or may not be related to your diabetes. Many sexual problems can be treated once their cause is identified. So don't suffer in silence. Discuss the difficulty with your physician.

sick days
(SIK DAZE)

The common cold, the flu, and other illnesses can present special problems for you if you have diabetes. Just the stress of illness can raise your blood-glucose level. And the "side effects" of illness, such as loss of appetite or vomiting, can also disrupt your ability to control your blood glucose.

easy-to-eat foods

FOOD	AMOUNT (FOR 1 EXCHANGE)	APPROX. CALORIES
Starch/Bread Exchanges		
Bread—white, whole wheat	1 slice	80
white, whole wheat toasted	1 slice	80
Cereal, hot	½ cup	80
Crackers		
Saltines	6	80
Graham crackers	3 (2½ in.)	80
Ice cream (any flavor)	½ cup (1 starch, 2 fat exch.)	170
Ice milk (any flavor)	½ cup (1 starch, 1 fat exch.)	125
Pudding (sugar-free, made with skim milk)	½ cup	80
Sherbert (any flavor)	¼ cup	80
Soups		
Vegetable or broth	1 cup (8 oz.)	80
Cream type (made with water)	1 cup (1 starch, 1 fat)	125
Meat Exchanges		
Cottage cheese	¼ cup	55
Egg Substitute (those with less than 55 calories per ¼ cup)	¼ cup	55
Egg Substitute (those with 55-80 calories per ¼ cup)	¼ cup	75
Egg, soft cooked or poached	1	75
Vegetable Exchanges		
Tomato juice	½ cup	25
Vegetable juice	½ cup	25

If you have insulin-dependent (type I) diabetes, you will probably need at least as much insulin as normal—even if you eat less than usual. You may even need more. If your diabetes is usually controlled by oral medication or meal planning, you may need to take insulin while you are ill to compensate for the stress illness can cause.

If you take insulin, you have to have food in your system. Try to follow your meal plan as closely as possible. If you feel too sick, though, switch to bland foods or liquids. If you can't stand having too much at one time, have a few sips of a non-diet soft drink or a few spoonfuls of pudding or the like and repeat about every 15 to 30 minutes.

The best approach to handling illness is to be prepared in advance with a sick-day plan. This should help you avoid hospitalization for diabetic coma (ketoacidosis). Agree on the plan with your doctor now and be sure that you have 24-hour, seven-day-a-week phone access to a physician should you need care.

Your sick-day plan will include guides for altering your insulin or pills, good food alternatives, changes in testing procedures, and any other information your doctor believes is necessary.

skiing
(SKEE-ing)

Brrrr. . .Crunch, Crunch, Crunch. . .Swoosh. . .Whee! What is all this? Why, they are the sounds of you skiing. Sure, just because you have diabetes doesn't mean you can't ski. In fact, skiing is a fun way of getting some exercise, and exercise is important to diabetes control.

Of course, people on the slopes who have diabetes must take more precautions than just making sure their bindings are tight. If you want to feel yourself slicing through a cool wind on a snowy mountain, follow this advice: Always carry identification that says you have diabetes. If you have an acci-

FOOD	AMOUNT (FOR 1 EXCHANGE)	APPROX. CALORIES
Fruit Exchanges		
Fruit juice		
cranberry juice cocktail, grape juice, and prune juice	⅓ cup	60
Apple juice/cider, grapefruit, orange, and pineapple	½ cup	60
Applesauce (unsweetened)	½ cup	60
Milk Exchanges		
Yogurt—plain, nonfat	8 oz.	90
Yogurt—plain, lowfat with added nonfat milk solids	1 cup (8 oz.)	120
Warm milk—skim	1 cup	90
Warm milk—½ percent	1 cup	90
Warm milk—1 percent	1 cup	90
Warm milk—2 percent	1 cup	120
Warm milk—whole	1 cup	150
Fat Exchanges		
Margarine	1 tsp.	45
Margarine (diet)	1 tbsp.	45
Free foods		
(less than 20 calories per serving)		
Fat-free broth or bouillon		
Black Coffee		
Tea		

skin

dent, the medics will know how to treat you. Also, it has been suggested that insulin is absorbed quickest from those body areas that are going to be active. So before skiing, you may want to inject in areas other than your legs, arms, or even your rear end if you fall a lot. Better than changing the site of insulin injections, however, is to wait at least 45 to 60 minutes after injecting before starting to exercise. See what your doctor has to say about injecting and exercise.

Be sure to let someone you are skiing with know about your diabetes and how to treat it should you have a reaction. Finally, carry food with you. Although you may, in fact, need to cut back on your insulin dosage if you exercise a lot, insulin reactions are still a possibility. Keep some crackers, peanut butter, and fast-acting carbohydrates (hard candy, a sugar packet) with you.

There now. Aren't you ready to attack the slopes? Just find yourself a mountain, snap on a pair of skis, and grab your poles. You're afraid of going down the slopes? Well, try cross-country skiing. It's usually cheaper, will give you a good aerobic workout, and you can stay on level ground.

skin
(SKIN)

We have heard a lot lately about what the sun can do to our skin, but did you know that diabetes can affect your skin, too? Of course, good control is important to keeping skin problems from occurring. And catching these problems before they get worse is all-important.

Here are some of the most common skin disorders associated with diabetes:

■ Bacterial infections. These usually occur as styes (infections of the glands and eyelids), boils, carbuncles, or inflammations around the nails. Staphylococcus ("staph") infections are particularly common. While these infections used to be life-threatening, antibiotics now make them relatively harmless.

■ Fungal infections. These are itchy rashes that usually occur in the moist areas of skin folds, such as the groin and armpits. Again, prescription medication can generally provide relief. Compresses of half a tablespoon of vinegar to a quart of water may also help.

■ Localized itching. Sometimes caused by a yeast infection, itching may also result from dry skin or poor circulation—both of which contribute to infections.

To help prevent such problems, avoid excessive bathing, use super-fatted soaps (such as Dove or Keri), practice careful hygiene, and report any inflammation to your physician, to help avoid serious skin infection problems.

When diabetes directly causes skin disorders, it often does so by causing changes in the blood vessels that supply the skin with nutrients, oxygen, and moisture. Two examples are *diabetic dermopathy* and *necrobiosis lipoidica diabeticorum*. Both of these cause small brown scaly patches on the shins. The first one is common but causes no pain and requires no treatment. The second one is fairly rare, which is fortunate

because the spots can be itchy and painful. Some ulcerate (break open), and if this happens, you should see your doctor as soon as possible.

Other skin problems, such as allergic reactions, can occur from oral medications or insulin injections. In particular, if you develop rashes, pits, or bumps at insulin-injection sites, see your doctor.

Two rare skin conditions can occur in people whose diabetes is out of control—diabetic blisters and eruptive xanthomatosis (small red bumps with yellow centers). The best treatment for these conditions is to bring diabetes under control. Sometimes prescription medicines that lower blood lipids are necessary.

If you do have skin problems, a dermatologist (skin specialist) may be better able to treat you than your regular doctor. Ask your doctor to refer you to one. Most dermatologists are familiar with the problems that may appear in people with diabetes.

smoking
(SMOKE-ing)

It's never too late to quit. Smoking is unhealthy for everybody. It can cause chronic bronchitis, emphysema, and lung cancer. Smoking has been shown to increase susceptibility to heart disease, and statistics show that smokers have a 70 percent higher risk of heart attacks than nonsmokers.

But for people with diabetes, the effects can be even worse. Since diabetes also contributes to heart disease, the odds are far worse for the smoker with diabetes. Also, both diabetes and smoking thicken small blood vessels, causing circulation problems that could ultimately lead to amputation.

Kicking the habit is tough, but the rewards are worth it. Just hours after you've put down your last cigarette, the nicotine begins to clear from your system and your body begins to heal. Within a few days, your sense of smell returns, and food starts to taste good again. Best of all, you feel more clear-headed, energetic, and *alive*.

The U.S. Department of Health and Human Services offers the following tips for cutting down:

■ Switch to a brand you dislike, best of all one that is low in tar and nicotine. If you enjoy the cigarettes less, you'll smoke less.

■ Smoke only half of each cigarette.

■ Wait until one pack is empty before buying another one, and never buy cigarettes by the carton.

■ Put cigarettes in an out-of-the-way place so you'll be more aware of each cigarette you smoke.

■ Don't empty the cigarette butts from your ashtray. Let the pile remind you of how many you've smoked in a day.

Once you've cut down and you're physically less dependent on tobacco, it will be much easier to stop entirely. On the day you quit:

■ Throw away all cigarettes and matches.

■ Begin to set aside the money you save on cigarettes to buy something special for yourself or someone else.

■ Keep busy; find activities that are incompatible with

smoking. Avoid situations, such as cocktail parties, where you might be tempted to smoke.

■ Do something to celebrate your quitting.

■ Brush your teeth often and use mouthwash to get used to having a clean taste in your mouth.

■ If you miss having something in your mouth, try a toothpick or a fake cigarette.

Many people find "stop-smoking" groups helpful because they provide social pressure and encouragement. Contact your local chapter of the American Cancer Society or the American Heart Association to find out about such groups in your area.

spices
(SPY-sez)

The average person has 10,000 taste buds, and one of the joys of eating is using them all! Because spices add exotic flavors to food, learning to use them can be an adventure. It can also help you cut calories by cutting out other, more caloric, flavorings such as butter or margarine, sour cream, gravies, sauces, nuts, and seeds.

Here are some spices and dishes to try them in:

■ Chili powder—corn, bean casseroles, cheese, marinades, chicken, meat loaf, stews, egg dishes, tomato or barbeque dishes, and dips.

■ Cinnamon—lamb and beef stews, roast lamb, chicken, pork, ham, beverages, bakery products, and fruit.

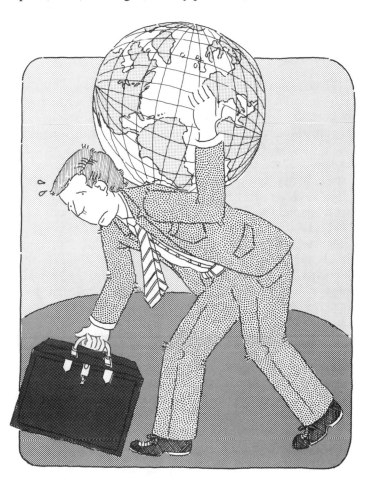

■ Curry powder—curried meat, poultry, and fish dishes, eggs, dried beans, fruit, dips, breads, salad dressings, and marinades.

■ Garlic—meat, poultry, fish, stews, marinades, tomato dishes, dips, sauces, salads, and salad dressings.

■ Ginger—baked or stewed fruits, vegetables, baked goods, poultry, fish, meat, beverages, soups, and many Oriental dishes.

■ Mint—sauces for lamb and poultry, punches, tea, sauces for desserts, and vegetables.

■ Mustard Seed—corned beef, coleslaw, potato salad, boiled cabbage, pickles, and sauerkraut.

■ Oregano—fish, meat, poultry, all vegetables, stuffings, cheese dishes, egg dishes, barbeque sauces, chili, pizza, pasta sauces, and tomatoes.

■ Paprika—fish, meat, poultry, egg and cheese dishes; adds color to colorless vegetables; sprinkle on casseroles for garnish.

■ Sage—stuffings for meats, fish, and poultry, sauces, soups, chowders, marinades, onions, tomatoes, and egg and cheese dishes.

starch/bread exchange list
(STARCH/BRED eks-CHANJ LIST)

We're not just talking a slice of bread and a potato here. This list includes such things as grits, waffles, pretzels, popcorn, baked beans, bread sticks and bagels. There are six categories within the Starch/Bread Exchange list. They include: cereals, grains, and pasta; dried beans, peas, and lentils; starchy vegetables; bread; crackers and snacks; and starch foods prepared with fat.

Each item on the Starch/Bread list contains approximately 15 grams of carbohydrate, 3 grams of protein, a trace of fat, and 80 calories. Many items on this list are complex carbohydrates. (Some complex carbohydrates are found in foods such as bread, pasta, cereal, rice, and beans.) These are good for a person with diabetes because they take longer to break down in digestion and cause a more gradual increase in blood sugar (see Carbohydrates).

For a more complete listing of this exchange group, check a copy of the American Diabetes Association's *Exchange Lists for Meal Planning*.

stress
(STRESS)

Stress can be hazardous to your health! But how can you avoid it? You can't. We are all under stress *all* the time. The stress you experience may be minor—such as forgetting to put a dime in a parking meter and worrying that you may get a ticket—or it can be rather serious—such as fear that you will be unable to find a new job when your company moves away.

sugar

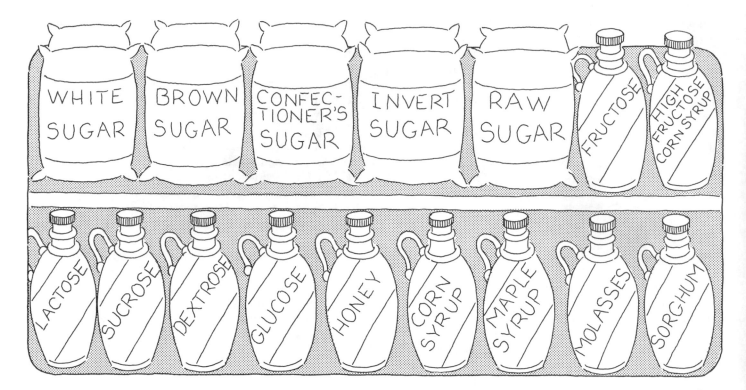

These two examples are instances of psychological stress. You can also experience physical stress—this results from such things as illness, infections, overexercised muscles, or fever.

Stress is a body reaction. A change in your environment—physical or psychological—can set off a secretion (release) of hormones that can provide your muscles and nervous system with energy that they need to react fast. These hormones can be invaluable in life-threatening situations because they help you make urgent decisions and act quickly.

But if you are constantly under stress, your body gets charged up and has no way to channel all that energy. The result can be physically debilitating. Signs of excessive stress include stomach upset or headaches, diarrhea, rashes, coughing, depression, fatigue, and elevated blood glucose.

Stress makes your blood sugar rise because that is the role of one of the stress-related hormones—the sugar is supposed to be used for energy. If you don't have enough insulin to handle the stress, or the insulin isn't effective, the sugar will build up in your blood. This buildup can ruin your control if the stress is severe enough.

Because this is the case, you will want to try to remove some of the stress factors from your life, or at least change your thoughts about them. If some of your stress is related to your job and is predictable (such as meeting deadlines), maybe some better planning and organizational habits will help you eliminate some of the stress. Learning to cope with stress as it happens is important. When you feel a lot of stress, try to calm down and relax. If you're at home, you might want to lie on your couch, close your eyes, and relax with some quiet, soft music. (See Relaxation.) Besides helping to keep your diabetes in control, regular exercise may also help you deal with stress better. Your doctor may also be able to give you some helpful ideas on how to relieve some of the stress in your

life. Or your doctor may be able to refer you to a psychologist or social worker who specializes in helping people manage stress.

sugar
(SHOOG-er)

There is an old myth that people with diabetes should avoid all sugars. This is neither true nor realistic. The *regular* use of concentrated sugar should be avoided because sugar is absorbed quickly into the bloodstream, causing a rise in blood glucose. Concentrated sugars are found in such foods as jams, jellies, pastries, ice cream, cookies, cakes, pies, candy, honey, syrup, and soft drinks. You cannot avoid *all* sugar because many basic foods such as bread, milk, and fruit, contain small amounts of sugar. These foods are included in your daily meal plan in order to provide a balanced nutritional diet. Also, if you work it into your meal plan, you may be able to eat foods containing small amounts of sugar occasionally. Of course, you need to take sugar or sugary foods when you have an insulin reaction. You just need to avoid overtreating the reaction by eating more than you need.

Sugar is a nutritive sweetner, meaning it contains calories. Nutritive sweeteners are sugars such as white, brown, confectioner's, invert, and raw; fructose; high-fructose corn syrup; lactose; sucrose, dextrose, and glucose; honey; corn syrup; maple syrup; molasses; and sorghum. Familiarize yourself with the many names by which sugar is known, read labels carefully, and avoid processed foods that are high in sugar.

You *may* be able to incorporate a touch of sugar into your

meal plan for an occasional treat—if your diabetes and weight are in good control. But you will need to do careful monitoring. Ask your diet counselor for advice.

sugar substitutes
(SHOOG-er SUB-stah-toots)

Do you ever wish you could eat sugar and not suffer from the extra calories or high blood sugar? Yes, that would be great, but it just ain't so. Fortunately, there is the next best thing—sugar substitutes.

These sweeteners may not completely match the taste of sugar, but they are an alternative, if you are having trouble keeping sugar out of your meal plan. Besides the fact that these sweeteners do not completely resemble sugar, there is some controversy concerning their safety. The decision to use sugar substitutes is up to you depending on your overall diet and nutritional needs. Of course, you should discuss this with your doctor or dietitian, but we thought you might appreciate a little information on different sweeteners being used today.

■ Aspartame: This sweetener is considered nutritive (meaning it contains calories), but because it is 180 to 220 times sweeter than sugar, the amount you would use would have virtually no calories. It is a man-made sweetener made from aspartic acid and phenylalanine, two of the amino acids found in proteins. (People with phenylketonuria (PKU) should not use aspartame.) Moderate use of aspartame is approved by the American Diabetes Association.

■ Saccharin: This sweetener has no calories. It has been found that high doses of saccharin have caused bladder cancer in some laboratory animals. However, scientific research has found no evidence that saccharin causes cancer in humans. Of course, the threat of cancer can't be ruled out. The risk of getting cancer from moderate use of this sweetener is extremely small. The American Diabetes Association also approves the use of saccharin. However, if you are pregnant, you should avoid heavy use of saccharin. This sweetener can be passed from mother to baby.

■ Acesulfame-K: This sweetener also has no calories. Its big advantage is that it can be used for baking because it is not destroyed by high heat. Except for containing a small amount of potassium, it is somewhat similar in makeup to saccharin, so follow the guidelines for use of saccharin.

■ Fructose: This sweetener contains calories, but does not raise blood sugar significantly in people with well-controlled diabetes. Fructose is not recommended for use by people whose diabetes is poorly controlled because it does cause a rapid blood-sugar rise in them. When used in cold or acidic foods, it is about twice as sweet as table sugar. For this reason, you can sometimes get the same sweetness as sugar with half the calories. *Fructose is not recommended for people with diabetes who are trying to lose weight because it does contain calories.*

■ Sorbitol, Mannitol, Xylitol: These three are sugar alcohols found in many plants and are sometimes used by manufacturers as sweeteners. The long-term effects of these substitutes are not known. However, they can be harmful because they can cause diarrhea when eaten in large amounts (more than an ounce in a day). They are also not useful in weight-loss because they contain calories.

support groups
(sah-PORT GROOPS)

Support groups come in all shapes and sizes, but all share the same basic premise: Sharing your feelings with people who have the same concerns as you helps to combat loneliness, gives you new ideas for coping, and opens the way to new friendships.

There are diabetes support groups for teens, parents,

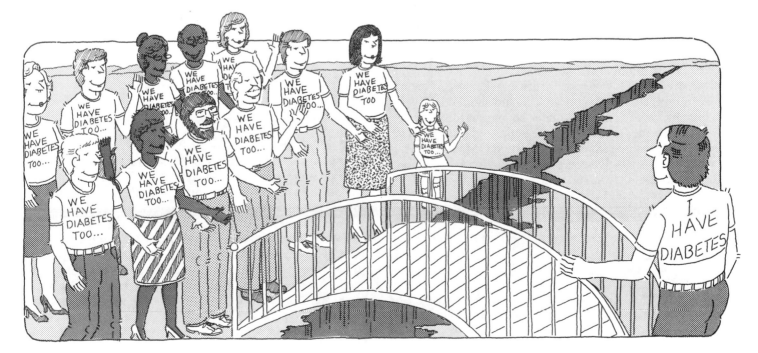

swimming

overweight people, spouses, and people with complications. To find out about support groups near you, contact your American Diabetes Association chapter or affiliate. If the type of group you need does not exist, discuss starting one. If you have a need, chances are others near you do, too.

swimming
(SWIM-ming)

Throughout this publication, we have emphasized the importance of exercise in relation to maintaining good diabetes control. We admit that exercise is not always fun, nor is it easy to get in the habit of a regular routine. But maybe—just maybe—we have found an exercise you can easily jump into—literally (providing the water isn't too cold).

Swimming is great for your body. The water can soothe your body and give your muscles a great workout at the same time. If done vigorously, swimming is a good form of aerobic activity—and that's good news for your heart and lungs. As opposed to many other aerobic exercises, swimming isn't bone-jarring and hard on your legs and feet, thus you are freer from injuries.

Many public pools offer a variety of swimming classes. There are water aerobics classes, hydrocalisthenics, and arthritis water exercise classes. Check out your local pool for more information. It might be a good idea to observe a class before signing up to see if it is for you. If you can, talk to people in the class to see if they find the class beneficial. Find out who the best instructor is.

Of course, before you dive into any exercise routine, check with your doctor first. If you decide on a class, let your instructor know you have diabetes. Inform your instructor about diabetes and how to treat an insulin reaction, just in case. One of the American Diabetes Association pamphlets, such as *What You Need to Know About Diabetes*, might be a good source of information for him or her. Be sure to bring a quick-acting carbohydrate (such as hard candy, orange juice, or a sugar packet) with you to leave at the edge of the pool. Before jumping in, check your blood-glucose level. If it is above 250 mg/dl, check your urine for ketones. If ketones are present, you need more insulin and should delay your swim until your diabetes is under better control.

OK, grab your towel, your nose plug, goggles, and splash away. And just one more word of advice: Make sure your bathing suit is tightly secured before diving in—you don't want to shock everyone on your first day.

tax tips
(TAKS TIPS)

As April 15th approaches each year, many people find themselves in a panic trying to get their taxes done on time. If this time of year pushes your nerves over the edge, you might want to turn to the section on stress. But before you do, let's try and relieve some of your worries: Some of your diabetes care may be deductible.

Unfortunately, because the tax laws change from time to time, it makes it difficult for us to be too specific. And before you dream of dollar-for-dollar tax returns, remember that your medical expenses will have to exceed a certain percentage of your adjusted gross income. (To get any of these deductions, you will have to itemize on your tax form.) We want to at least expose you to some possible deductions that relate to diabetes. Then you should check with your tax advisor to see how you can meet these deductions, if at all.

First, be sure to keep all receipts and a record of your medical and diabetes care expenses. You may be able to deduct your medical insurance premiums and your diabetes supplies. Keep receipts of everything you buy: insulin, oral diabetes medications, testing strips, cotton balls, alcohol swabs, and disposable syringes.

Also, keep track of things not covered by insurance. For instance, travel to the doctor, hospital, and pharmacist for treatment and supplies for your diabetes may be deductible. The cost of belonging to a diabetes support group may be deductible. If your doctor has advised you to join a weight-loss program, that too might be deductible. Treatment for mental health is also generally deductible.

We hope we have given you something to think about. Your best bet now is to discuss these deductions with your tax advisor and plan for the next year.

Still feel stressed out? Besides the section on stress, you might check the section on exercise, too—not only is exercise good for your diabetes control, it's a great way to relieve stress.

tight control
(tite kon-TROL)
See Control

transplants
(trans-PLANTS)

Wouldn't it be nice if an organ transplant could be as simple as putting together a child's toy? Just imagine: "Insert pancreas A into abdomen B and discard insulin supplies." That would be wonderful. But unfortunately, the process is much more complicated than that.

If you were to have a pancreas transplant performed, you would be faced with certain risks. Besides the surgery itself, a big risk of transplantation is rejection. Your body may reject the new pancreas because it recognizes it as foreign. Your body's immune system may repeat what it did to *your* pancreas and destroy the beta (insulin-producing) cells in the new transplanted pancreas.

Rejection can sometimes be corrected with the use of

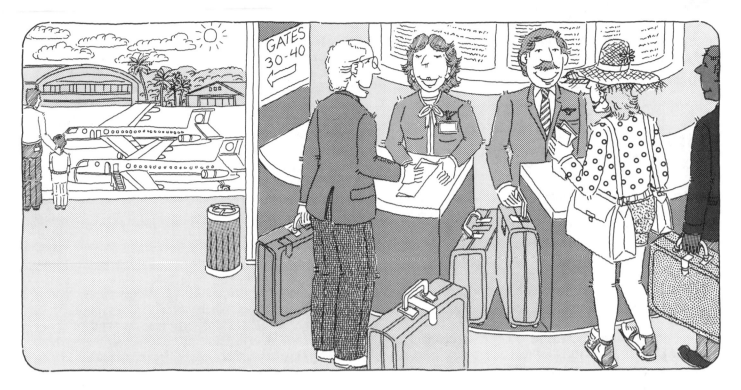

immunosuppressive drugs. These drugs reduce the body's ability to attack alien substances. The problem with these medications is that they can increase a person's risk of developing infections.

There is also another type of transplant being studied—that of the islet cells that produce insulin. Rather than removing the whole pancreas, this process would "repair" the existing one. However, like the pancreas itself, these cells can be rejected, too. Scientists are working to find a way to prevent this rejection. They have had promising results in animals, but have yet to be successful in humans. Because transplantation of islet cells is safer and easier than that of the pancreas itself, this may be the way of the future—if the problems of rejection and of getting the islet cells to continue producing insulin over the long term can be overcome.

travel

(TRAV-l)

Thinking of traveling somewhere for your vacation but don't know if you should because you have diabetes? Well, stop worrying and get packing. All traveling with diabetes means is you have to take a few extra preparations and precautions. Perhaps the following tips will come in handy:

To avoid the fatigue of crowds, you might want to travel in off-peak seasons. You will get better accommodations at a lower cost and find personnel in hotels, restaurants, and sightseeing spots more willing to spend time to meet your needs. For travel within the United States, contact your local American Diabetes Association for the number of an affiliate at your destination. If you are heading abroad, contact the International Diabetes Federation for names and addresses of local diabetes associations. Their address is 40 Rue Washington, 1050 Brussels, Belgium. Write ahead to find out about the availability of insulin and syringes by various manufacturers (in particular, the concentrations in which insulin is available), and discuss this information with your doctor. Such associations should be able to help you find an English-speaking doctor, if needed.

Before leaving on a long trip, be sure to see your physician for a checkup. He or she can offer advice on adjusting insulin doses and eating schedules as you cross time zones or otherwise alter your routine. Ask for a letter on letterhead explaining that you have diabetes and listing the medications you take. This will help if you have to explain why you are carrying syringes through customs. Get a prescription for syringes and needles in case a pharmacist demands one.

Plan to take along a more-than-adequate supply of any prescription drugs you need. It may also help to have your doctor give you an extra prescription that has the generic (general) name of the drug you use to help aid understanding in a foreign country.

When you are packing, stash all diabetes supplies in bags that you will keep with you at all times. When flying, never store drugs in luggage headed for the baggage compartment. Not only might it wind up at a different destination, but medicine may be destroyed by temperature extremes in baggage compartments. In your "carry-on" bag, pack extra food (such as cheese and crackers) to deal with delays, and some form of concentrated sugar (gels, sugar cubes) in case you become hypoglycemic.

If you don't already wear a medical ID bracelet or necklace that indicates you have diabetes, now is the time to invest in one. Keep additional health information on a card in your wallet, including your doctor's name and phone number.

type I/type II
(TIPE ONE/TIPE TWO)

See Diabetes

units
(YOO-nits)

When insulin first came into use, manufacturers, physicians, and insulin-users alike needed a way to measure it. Eventually, a standard quantity known as the insulin "unit" was developed. A unit of insulin is now defined as $1/24$th of a milligram of pure insulin.

The concentration or strength of an insulin formulation is measured in *units of insulin per milliliter of fluid*. U-100 insulin, for example, contains 100 units of insulin in each milliliter.

At one time, insulin was sold in a variety of concentrations, including U-10, U-20, U-40, U-80, and U-100. Now, however, all insulin concentrations except U-100 have been phased out in the United States. The reason is to avoid confusion and risk of getting the wrong dosage of insulin. The important thing to remember is: If you use U-100 insulin be sure you are using a U-100 syringe.

Syringes for different concentrations of insulin are graded differently. If you use a U-40 syringe for U-100 insulin, you will get more than twice the dosage you were expecting.

If you travel overseas, you may find that different unit measurements than those used in the United States are available. If you will be traveling outside the United States, you are better off bringing a supply of insulin and syringes with you (see Travel). The country you are visiting may not have insulin in the concentration you use. You should not change the concentration of insulin without your doctor's supervision. Again, if you do change, remember to use the right syringe with the proper unit of insulin.

Highly concentrated (such as U-500) insulin is also available for special situations. In general, most people never need it. It is also used for treating rare cases of extreme insulin resistance, in which a person needs to take very large doses of insulin in order for it to work properly.

urine tests
(YER-in TESTS)

There really is no substitute for blood tests when it comes to accurately monitoring your blood-glucose level. In the beginning, urine tests were the only way individuals with diabetes could monitor their control. But now, many people who have diabetes monitor their control by daily self-monitoring of blood glucose. That's because urine tests can only give a rough reading of blood-glucose levels. And a rough reading won't give you the information you need for tight control of your blood glucose.

The level of sugar in your urine is only a reflection of the actual levels in your blood. Urine tests only reflect *past* blood glucose levels—those levels that occurred several hours before the test was taken. Your blood glucose may be fine at the time of the test, but your urine test could "read" high because your blood sugar was high several hours before you tested. Also, a urine test can "read" negative for sugar, but your blood sugar could actually be low, normal, or even high. Sometimes, sugar can "spill" over into the urine. (The point at which sugar "spills over" into the urine is known as the *renal threshold*.) When this happens, a urine test may "read" high, but your actual blood-sugar level may be at normal levels between 80-140 mg/dl.

Does this mean you can stop testing your urine forever? *Absolutely not*. Urine tests provide vital information that can help you avoid ketoacidosis or diabetic coma. Testing your urine is the only way you can measure ketones (tiny fragments of fatty acids that appear when the body starts to burn its own stores of fat. See Ketoacidosis.) When your body is under serious stress—like a bad flu or intestinal upset—you may be producing too many ketone bodies. If you find ketones in your urine, you could be developing ketoacidosis, and you should quickly contact your doctor to discuss the situation.

There are a variety of urine tests on the market. Some test for both glucose and ketones. Some test only for one or the other. Tests vary in how you perform them and how you "read" the findings. You'll need to work with your doctor and nurse to find the kind of test that works best for you.

You should talk with your doctor about which test to use. Some are easier to read and some are more accurate than others. Find what works best for you.

Also, the decision of whether or not to use urine tests to measure glucose is something you and your doctor need to make. Some people use both blood and urine tests and find that the combination helps them to take even better control of their diabetes.

vaccines
(vak-SEENS)

While smallpox is not a threat to our health today, it was in the 18th century—20 percent of all deaths were caused by smallpox. This was until 1798 when Edward Jenner designed a vaccine for smallpox. This was the first vaccine ever developed. Since then, numerous vaccines have been developed to prevent diseases such as polio, tetanus, diphtheria, and the measles. But what exactly are vaccines and how do they affect a person who has diabetes?

Vaccines contain small amounts of deactivated microorganisms that in their natural form can cause a disease. When your body gets a "taste" of the disease, it alerts your immune system to boost its defenses against the disease. Then if you come in contact with the "real thing," your body is armed and ready.

Vaccines, for the most part, are as safe for people with

diabetes as they are for anyone else. However, some people develop side effects to certain vaccines. When side effects, such as a slight fever, occur in people with diabetes, they can interfere with control. Normally, this isn't a major problem. But if you are planning an international vacation, don't leave vaccinations for the last minute. It is easier to cope with side effects and regain control on home turf.

What about the flu season? Should you get a vaccine or not? Doctors have differing opinions on this. However, many agree that people with diabetes, particularly the elderly, are at special risk when they get the flu. For this reason, elderly people especially should be vaccinated before the flu season begins (usually around early fall). Once the flu sets in, it can disrupt diabetes control severely and your body may have difficulty fighting the infection. (See Sick Days.) Elderly people, especially, may develop severe complications of the flu such as pneumonia. For this reason, it might also be a good idea to get vaccinated against pneumonia, too. You can get both flu and pneumonia shots at the same time. However, while flu shots can be given every year, shots for pneumonia should be given only once.

Our advice? Check with your doctor and discuss the best approach you can take to prevent getting sick. Your doctor can help you determine or monitor the effects a vaccine can have on you.

vegetable exchange list
(VEJ-tah-bal eks-CHANJ LIST)

Mom was right—you need to eat your vegetables. Besides being a great source of fiber, vegetables are also a good way to get many of the vitamins and minerals you need.

The Vegetable exchange list gives you a choice of vegetables to enjoy. However, you may be surprised that some of the vegetables you like, such as corn and peas, are not on the list. If you don't find your favorites on this list, you might want to check the Starch/Bread exchange list. Many vegetable choices are also listed in the Free Food section.

Now, eat all your vegetables or there is no TV tonight! Sorry, we just thought you might need a little push. It worked for Mom, didn't it?

vegetarianism
(VEJ-ah-TARE-ee-ahn-izm)

There was a day when many people not only thought vegetarians were nuts, but that they were also full of baloney. But with today's knowledge about the health threats of excessive fatty animal flesh and the benefits of vegetables and whole grains, more people are incorporating this food style into their meal plans.

True vegetarians consume *only* plant foods and eliminate all animal products. They get protein solely from legumes—

such as dried peas, beans and lentils—and grains. Meeting your nutritional needs on such a diet can be difficult, but that's only one of the various approaches. Some vegetarians use the "lacto-ovo" approach in the vegetarian diet. This approach includes dairy products (milk, cheese, butter, yogurt) and eggs.

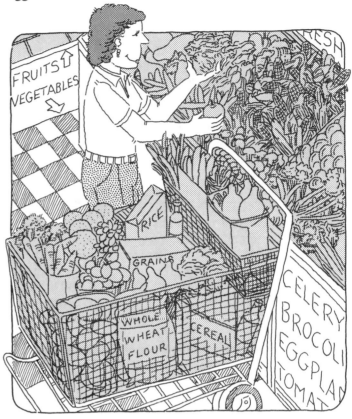

But you don't have to become a total vegetarian to reap the benefits of vegetarianism. Americans, in general, eat too much meat. If your meal plans are centered around meat, you may want to consider altering your meals to include more starches and vegetables into your meal plans. By doing so, you will limit your intake of the fat in meat, which can contribute to heart disease. Also, the vegetarian diet tends to be bulkier because the calories in grains and vegetables are less concentrated than those in meat. That's good news because it means you can eat more food for the same number of calories. Because you will feel full sooner, a vegetarian diet may help you lose weight. Vegetarians tend to weigh less and have lower blood cholesterol levels than nonvegetarians. Finally, your total food costs will be lower when you limit expensive meats.

You may also find an extra bonus: For some people, eating a vegetarian diet high in complex carbohydrates and fiber may actually decrease their insulin requirement. This is because a diet high in complex carbohydrates helps to slow the rise in blood sugar.

Thinking of converting totally to vegetarianism? Be sure to discuss it with your doctor and dietitian first. While a strictly vegetarian diet may be perfect for you, there may be some specific guidelines you will need to follow to meet your nutritional needs and to keep your diabetes in control.

viruses

viruses
(VI-rus-es)

Can a viral infection trigger insulin-dependent (type I) diabetes? That idea was first published in medical literature in the 1800s, and researchers today still believe this is possible. They have observed that type I diabetes sometimes follows a viral infection. Some viral infections under suspicion are the flu, mumps, and Coxsackie.

Researchers are still trying to unravel the complex events that lead to diabetes and the role they may play. Thus far, it looks like there is a three-step process to getting the disease:

■ First, you have to inherit a certain combination of genes that can make you susceptible to diabetes. These genes affect the nature of certain antigens. The antigens are part of the body's immune system. They spot and destroy such invaders as bacteria and viruses. (Antigens are actually proteins that sit on cells throughout the body, including the insulin-producing beta cells of the pancreas.)

■ Second, a virus invades the system and interacts with body cells. How these interactions occur is still unknown.

■ Third, the beta cells are destroyed—although how this happens is not clearly known. One possibility is that the immune system does not fight off the viruses well enough. This allows the viruses to enter the beta cells and destroy them directly. Another theory is that the immune system overreacts—acting as if the body's own beta cells were foreign invaders—and destroys the beta cells. This is known as an *autoimmune response.* (Stress may also trigger the autoimmune response in people.)

As scientists learn more about these processes, they may be able to develop vaccines to prevent viral infection, or antiviral agents to stop viruses from growing. But they will have to identify many genes and many more viruses before that day comes.

vision
(VIZH-un)

Spotting eye problems early is the key to maintaining good vision. In addition to diabetic retinopathy, there are a number of other vision problems that all people, not just those with diabetes, may face. If caught in time, most of them can be corrected.

Focusing difficulties that come and go are a classic sign of undiagnosed diabetes. A person may have excellent vision one day, be quite nearsighted the next, and then have normal vision when visiting the doctor another day. As soon as blood glucose is regulated, the eye generally settles down and operates well, though the problem can recur if diabetes gets out of control.

Cataracts, when they occur, may develop slightly earlier in people with diabetes than in others. One of the symptoms of cataracts is blurred vision. People with cataracts may also have the impression that pieces are missing from the image they see, or they may see double or see halos when looking into lights. While there is no proven way to prevent cataracts or other eye diseases, experts agree that good diabetes control will help delay, if not prevent, them from occurring. If you do get cataracts, surgical treatment may restore vision if the cataract was the main block to seeing.

Although glaucoma (the buildup of fluid and pressure in the eye) does not appear to be caused by diabetes directly, people with diabetes are somewhat more likely to develop it. Its symptoms include no improvement in vision after an eyeglass prescription is changed, headaches after watching TV or movies, difficulty focusing in a darkened room, and seeing halos, colored rings, or rainbows around lights. Glaucoma may be prevented from causing blindness if detected early and treated with eyedrops or pills that decrease fluid in the eye.

One other vision problem is neuropathy. This happens when one of the small muscles that move the eye becomes temporarily paralyzed, because of damage to the nerve that controls it. The result is pain and double vision. This form of neuropathy is rare and generally improves without treatment.

Your eyesight is too valuable to be lost to improper care. Be sure to have an ophthalmic exam at least once a year, or more regularly if your doctor advises. Consult your eye doctor immediately if you have any vision problems. Being on the lookout for eye problems can save your sight.

vitamins
(VIT-ah-mins)

Some people wonder if vitamin supplements will help their diabetes. The answer? We don't know. Some health professionals favor vitamin supplements, while others do not. Some just leave the decision up to you.

Ideally, if you follow your meal plan, you will get all the nutrients you need. But let's face it, we don't always eat the way we should.

Should *you* take vitamins? There is certainly no harm in taking one multiple vitamin a day, and it may benefit your health. However, don't take large amounts of vitamins—some tend to build up in the body and can be toxic (poisonous) in large doses (for example, vitamins A and D). Vitamins with iron or zinc may also be harmful to you. Ask you doctor before taking them.

Remember that vitamins are *not* substitutes for good food. Fiber, protein, and other essential nutrients are found only in food—and in larger quantities in unprocessed than in processed foods.

Some processed foods may have vitamins added to them. If the vitamins are ones that are a natural part of the food's ingredients, the food is said to be *vitamin enriched* (often done to replace vitamins destroyed during processing). If, as is often done in breakfast cereals, vitamins are added that do not naturally occur in the ingredients, the food is said to be *vitamin fortified.* While most dietitians see no great harm in enrichment or fortification, they do stress that vitamins alone do not a good food make.

One final point: Vitamins—regardless of the dosage—cannot cure diabetes.

walking
(WAHK-ing)

If you don't like the bone-jarring stress running puts on your joints and muscles, you might consider walking to get your aerobic exercise.

A regular fitness program where you walk vigorously for 20 to 30 minutes several days a week has many benefits. You can condition your heart and lungs, and the muscles in your arms, abdomen, legs, and lower back. Also, a regular walking program can help you reduce fat and may help your body use insulin more efficiently.

Walking is probably the safest aerobic exercise there is. However, like all exercise programs, first check with your doctor. You may have a physical condition that may prevent you from benefiting from a strenuous walking program. Also, be sure to wear a good pair of shoes. If you can, get a pair of "walking shoes," as opposed to "running shoes." Walking shoes have a curved sole that aids the movement of the entire foot from heel to toe.

When you have diabetes, you need to take extra precautions. If your blood-glucose level is above 250 mg/dl, you should check your urine for ketones. If the test is positive for ketones, you need more insulin and should delay your exercise routine until you get your glucose closer to normal levels and are free of ketones. If your glucose is abnormally high, exercise may make it worse because there is not enough insulin in your blood to properly lower it.

If you take insulin, always carry a fast-acting carbohydrate such as hard candy or a sugar pack. If you notice early signs of hypoglycemia coming on, treat it immediately. Don't wait until you get home to treat it.

After your walk, inspect your feet carefully. Look for injuries you may not have felt during your walk. This is really important if you have neuropathy because you could injure your foot without knowing it.

Also, remember to build up your endurance gradually. Don't expect to walk 20 minutes your first day. You can do more harm than good by overdoing it. Don't expect too much too soon, either. It takes time before you will notice any big changes such as toned muscles and improved cardiovascular fitness.

warning signs
(WARN-ing SINES)

"Diabetes. . . .that's the disease where people don't have enough sugar in the blood, right? But then how come you can't ever eat sugar?" There may well have been a time when you weren't sure of the answer yourself. It's understandable that people who don't have to deal with diabetes on a daily basis may have trouble understanding what diabetes is.

If you have insulin-dependent diabetes, your family and co-workers need to know the differences between the two principal medical emergencies you might face—insulin reac-

tions and ketoacidosis. We have included a chart that will help explain these differences. Keep it handy both at home and at work. Also, teach the people close to you how to treat an insulin reaction. Keep a supply of concentrated sugar (such as hard candy or a nondiet soft drink) handy to give you if you show signs of an insulin reaction. And, teach them that if you are unable to swallow they need to get you to the hospital. The people closest to you should also know how to inject glucagon in case you become unconscious (see Glucagon).

Also explain that if there is some doubt about the kind of problem you are experiencing, it is best to assume that it is an insulin reaction. Point out that a person can do more harm by *not* treating an insulin reaction than by giving sugar to someone who, in fact, is going through ketoacidosis. Of course, if the problem does turn out to be ketoacidosis, the only proper first aid is a quick trip to the hospital.

warning signs

KETOACIDOSIS (Diabetic Coma)		HYPOGLYCEMIC REACTION (Insulin Reaction)
Gradual	◄ ONSET ►	Sudden
Flushed, dry	◄ SKIN ►	Pale, moist
Drowsy	◄ BEHAVIOR ►	Excited, nervous, irritable, confused
Fruity odor (acetone)	◄ BREATH ►	Normal
Deep, labored	◄ BREATHING ►	Normal to rapid shallow
Present	◄ VOMITING ►	Absent
Dry	◄ TONGUE ►	Moist, numb, tingling
Absent	◄ HUNGER ►	Present
Present	◄ THIRST ►	Absent
High levels	◄ KETONES ►	Negligible
High	◄ GLUCOSE IN URINE ►	Low

weight loss
(WATE LOSS)

If you are overweight and have non-insulin-dependent (type II) diabetes, you have probably heard it all before: Lose weight, and your body will probably be able to use the insu-

xylitol

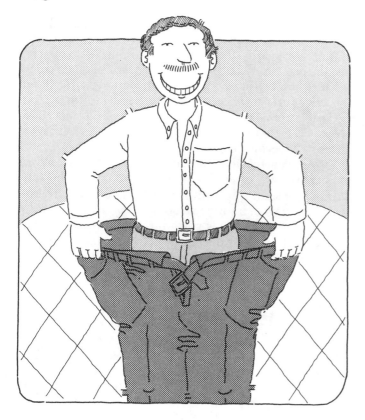

lin it produces more efficiently. If you use medication (whether insulin or oral diabetes medication), losing weight may also help you to cut down your dosage.

There is no secret to losing weight—it's a matter of taking in fewer calories than you burn up. Here are some suggestions to help you in your battle of the bulge:

■ Keep a food diary to help you become more aware of why you overeat. Record the time and what you were doing at the time. Were you watching TV or watching someone else eat? Also record your feelings at the time. Were you angry, bored, or sad? See if any pattern of overeating emerges from the diary.

■ Set reasonable goals for yourself. Weight reduction should be slow. Don't expect too much too soon. Weight reduction will happen gradually. Don't weigh yourself too often. It's easy to get discouraged if you don't see noticeable results on the scale. If you slip up and eat something you shouldn't, don't get discouraged and go on a real eating binge. That one slip-up likely won't affect your diet much. Just pick yourself up and get back on track.

■ Never go grocery shopping when you are hungry. You may be tempted to buy a lot of food you'll regret later. Write out a shopping list before you go to the market and stick to it.

■ Don't watch TV or listen to the radio while you're eating. Without these distractions, you'll feel you're getting more out of each mouthful.

■ Get involved in family projects or community activities. Many people eat out of boredom and find that other activities are more fulfilling.

■ Take up a new hobby. If you get involved in sewing or woodcrafting, for instance, your hands will be busy and your mind occupied. And you won't have as much time to think about eating.

■ Reward yourself for meeting short-term goals. The reward should have nothing to do with eating. Buy yourself some new clothes or go to a show.

■ Restrict your eating to one place. Don't take food into your bedroom or study. This will reduce the number of places you associate with eating.

■ Keep food out of sight. If you don't see it, you may not think about it or be tempted to nibble on what you see.

■ If you do get tempted, take a walk or do some kind of exercise instead of eating. Contrary to popular belief, exercise does not increase hunger. It has the added advantage of burning calories and decreasing insulin dosage. It also makes you feel good about yourself, something overeating never does.

xylitol
(ZI-la-tall)

This sugar alcohol is a caloric sweetener (four calories per gram) that should only be used with extreme caution. Large amounts of xylitol cause diarrhea, and some animal studies have indicated that steady use may be linked to the development of tumors. Because of the potential danger, some manufacturers have discontinued their use of xylitol. (See Sugar Substitutes.)

yoga
(YO-ga)

There's more to yoga than being tied up in knots. Yoga exercises are not the kind that get your heart pounding and blood

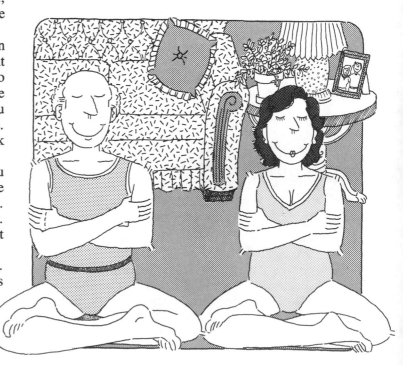

racing (see Exercise). In fact, they do just the opposite. Developed in India some 2,000 years ago, yoga has a relaxing, calming effect on both the mind and body and is an excellent stretching routine. Whatever your age or physical condition, you can probably benefit from yoga exercises. But be sure to check with your doctor before starting, just to make sure.

Yoga movements are not jarring, and, if taught and performed correctly, should never strain you or leave you feeling pained or exhausted. Yoga keeps muscles and joints flexible, improves circulation, and, in some cases, provides a gentle massage of internal organs, such as the intestines, which can aid regularity.

Perhaps most important, yoga reduces mental and physical tension. The pace of the yoga exercises is slow and controlled, with the various positions held for up to a minute. If you never stretch farther than feels totally comfortable, you are unlikely to ever have an injury from yoga. As an added benefit, yoga emphasizes deep-breathing techniques that help reduce stress. Once learned, these techniques can be used whenever you feel tense. (See Stress.)

To get started, pick up a book at your local library or a bookstore, or find a center that teaches yoga but won't demand that you sign up for a lifetime. Your local "Y" may offer a class. Keep in mind that most adults have lost a lot of the flexibility they once had; in general, women seem to be somewhat more flexible than men. It may take quite a while before you're really good at yoga, but don't give up. Even in the beginning stages, yoga is beneficial, and progress will come more quickly than you think. Yoga can be done throughout your life, and many people feel that the physical flexibility and strength they gain helps them maintain a youthful, positive attitude well into old age.

zest

(ZEST)

You peeked didn't you—you had to see what we came up with for the letter "z" before reading any of the other material. That's OK, because *Diabetes A to Z* is meant to be browsed through. Besides, maybe this is the best place to start since most of the information contained in this publication is designed to help you get that extra pizzazz from feeling good, the added determination to stay healthy, and the zest to live life to the fullest.

And how do you do that? Well, a big part of it is by keeping your diabetes under cont . . .wait a minute—we shouldn't tell you everything here. You're just going to have to back up and read the entries for Control, Exercise, Blood Testing, etc., for that answer. And we hope you'll study these pages with some zeal.

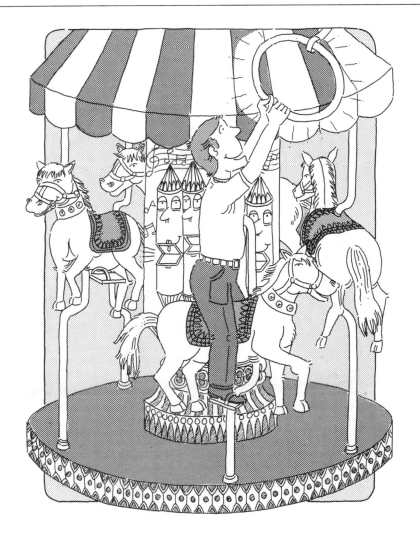

Index

Index

Meal planning made simple

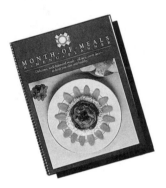

Month of Meals

Choose from 28 days' worth of breakfasts, lunches, and dinners that figure your calories and exchanges for you. There's also a selection of delicious snacks, and many of the menus have recipes, too! Plus step-by-step instructions for adapting the menus to different calorie levels.

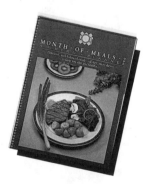

Month of Meals 2

Now there's another menu-planning book that can help you decide what to eat and how to fix it! Not only do you get a new choice of breakfasts, lunches, and dinners (28 days' worth), there are also tips on dining out at Mexican, Italian, Chinese, and fast food restaurants. Quick-to-fix and ethnic recipes are also included. Make meal planning automatic and enjoy *Month of Meals 2.*

Brand New!
Month of Meals 3

Your choices for breakfast, lunch, and dinner continue to grow with *Month of Meals 3*. Special sections include how to read ingredient labels on packages, meal planning for illness, and how to have picnics and barbecues and stay within your meal plan. High-fiber meals are also indicated. Available March 1992.

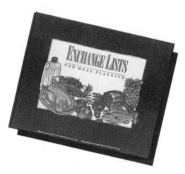

Exchange Lists for Meal Planning

Colorful charts, helpful tips on good nutrition, and the six easy-to-use food Exchange Lists show you how to balance your diet and gain control over diabetes. (Also available in large print.)

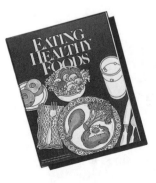

Eating Healthy Foods

This booklet provides daily food choices for breakfast, lunch, dinner, and snacks using the Exchange Lists.

Other ADA Publications

Healthy cooking that tastes great!

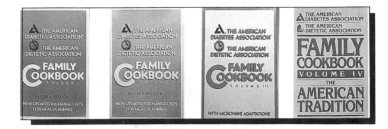

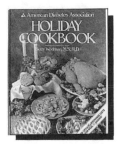

American Diabetes Association Holiday Cookbook

by Betty Wedman, M.S., R.D.

Enjoy the holidays more with recipes from traditional Thanksgiving, Christmas, and Hanukkah feasts . . . to savory meals for any occasion.

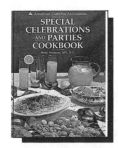

American Diabetes Association Special Celebrations and Parties Cookbook

by Betty Wedman, M.S., R.D.

Whether it's a Fourth of July barbecue, Mother's Day brunch, or birthday bash, these recipes invite everyone to join in.

Family Cookbook, Volume I

More than 250 delicious, economical, kitchen-tested recipes fill the pages of Volume I. It offers an encyclopedia of nutrition information, tips on eating out, brown-bagging, weight control, exercise, and much more.

Family Cookbook, Volume II

Volume II includes ways to cut sugar, calories, and costs—plus there are more than 250 tasty recipes! It has an entire section devoted to living with diabetes and gives advice on the emotional aspects of dieting.

Family Cookbook, Volume III

Add to your recipe treasury with more than 200 delicious recipes. Included are tips on microwaving, food processing, and freezing for fix-ahead meals. Recipes from various ethnic cuisines are included.

Brand New!
Family Cookbook, Volume IV, The American Tradition

Recipes from Boston Scrod to Santa Fe Chicken (more than 200 recipes in all) fill each page of this new cookbook with great American flavor. Volume IV also includes a colorful introductory section of interesting facts about the history of American cuisine.

For parents & kids

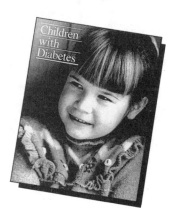

Children With Diabetes

Essential for parents, teachers, and others who work with diabetic children. It covers all the details of diabetes management, takes a sensitive look at children's psychological needs, and offers suggestions for promoting a positive and supportive home environment.

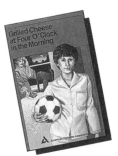

Grilled Cheese at Four O'Clock in the Morning

This unique children's novel presents vital information to your child by allowing him or her to identify with Scott, the main character in the book. In learning to cope with his diabetes, Scott learns some important lessons about himself—and life. Ages 8–12.

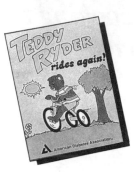

Teddy Ryder Rides Again!

A coloring book just for kids with diabetes. It's a story about Teddy Ryder, a young bear who develops diabetes. Let Teddy help your child learn more about the disease. Ages 3–8.

More about diabetes

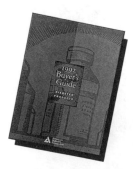

Brand New!
1992 Buyer's Guide to Diabetes Products

An excellent guide for comparing features from different manufacturers for everything from insulin, syringes, and jet injectors to insulin pumps, injection aids, test strips, and more.

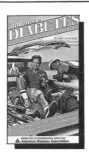

Diabetes: A Positive Approach—Video

Join Comedian Tom Parks, anchorman for HBO's ''Not Necessarily the News'' and National Chairman for the American Diabetes Association's Comedy Crusade Against Diabetes, in this unique video. You'll laugh as you learn to fit self-care into your active life.

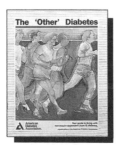

The 'Other' Diabetes

A thorough explanation of type II diabetes, this lively, colorful booklet provides practical advice as you learn how to live a happier, healthier life with proper treatment, diet, and exercise.

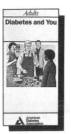

Diabetes and You: Adults

This popular ADA booklet is geared to dealing with your special needs, including complications, coping, care, and control. Also available is *Diabetes & You: Seniors*.

Especially for women

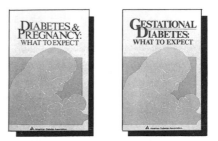

Diabetes & Pregnancy: What to Expect

The comprehensive guide for women with type I diabetes who are pregnant or are thinking about having a baby.

Gestational Diabetes: What to Expect

Here's the guide that helps you learn what gestational diabetes is and how to care for yourself during your pregnancy.

For people who want to know more

ADA Product Catalog

This new catalog details all the latest publications and products on diabetes from the ADA—for both the person with diabetes and the health-care team. Just indicate on your order that you want your own free copy.

Send your check or money order payable to:
American Diabetes Association
1970 Chain Bridge Road
McLean, VA 22109-0592

Allow 4–6 weeks for delivery. Add $3.00 to shipping & handling for each additional ''ship to'' address. Foreign orders must be paid in U.S. funds, drawn on a U.S. bank. Prices subject to change without notice.

Shipping & Handling Chart
up to $5.00 . . . . add $1.75
$5.01–$10.00 . . . . add $3.00
$10.01–$25.00 . . . . add $4.50
$25.01–$50.00 . . . . add $5.50
over $50.00 . . . . add 10% of order

To Order ADA Publications

	Price nonmember/member

Meal planning made simple

Month of Meals	$ 10.00/$ 9.00
Month of Meals 2	$ 10.00/$ 9.00
Month of Meals 3	$ 10.00/$ 9.00
Exchange Lists for Meal Planning	$ 1.30/$ 1.10
Exchange Lists for Meal Planning—Large Print	$ 2.50/$ 2.15
Eating Healthy Foods	$ 2.00/$ 1.70

Healthy cooking that tastes great!

Family Cookbook, Volume I	$ 19.95/$ 17.95
Family Cookbook, Volume II	$ 23.00/$ 20.70
Family Cookbook, Volume III	$ 23.00/$ 20.70
Family Cookbook, Volume IV	$ 23.00/$ 20.70
American Diabetes Association Holiday Cookbook	$ 19.95/$ 17.95
American Diabetes Association Special Celebrations and Parties Cookbook	$ 19.95/$ 17.95

For parents & kids

Children With Diabetes	$ 7.95/$ 7.15
Grilled Cheese at Four O'Clock in the Morning	$ 5.95/$ 5.35
Teddy Ryder Rides Again!	$ 1.95/$ 1.75

More about diabetes

1992 Buyer's Guide to Diabetes Products	$ 2.95/$ 2.65
Diabetes: A Positive Approach—Video	$ 19.95/$ 17.95
The 'Other' Diabetes	$ 2.95/$ 2.65
Diabetes and You: Adults	$ 1.50/$ 1.35
Diabetes and You: Seniors	$ 1.50/$ 1.35

Especially for women

Diabetes & Pregnancy: What to Expect	$ 7.25/$ 6.55
Gestational Diabetes: What to Expect	$ 7.25/$ 6.55

For people who want to know more

ADA Product Catalog	FREE